Miracle
SUPER
FOODS
That Heal

Dr. Tony O'Donnell, N. D.
Naturopathic Doctor

ROBERT D. REED PUBLISHERS • SAN FRANCISCO, CA

Robert D. Reed Publishers
750 La Playa Street, Suite 647
San Francisco, CA 94121
Phone: 650-994-6570 • Fax: -6579
Email: 4bobreed@msn.com
Web site: www.rdrpublishers.com

Editor and Book Designer: Linda Moulton Howe
Assistant Editors: Jim Schenkel and Pamela D. Jacobs, M.A.
Assistant Typesetter: Marilyn Yasmine Nader
Cover Designers: Julia A. Gaskill and Tasha Jackson

Book text is New Baskerville 11 point
with Charlemagne titles.

ISBN 1-885003-84-6

Library of Congress Catalogue Number: 2001088127

Produced and Printed in the United States of America

This book is dedicated to my father and mother who inspired me to be the best I could be. I love you, Mom and Dad.

This book is also dedicated to my brothers and sisters who showered me with love. To Jill, who passed away much too soon. And to Darien Israel, who is so very special and made it all possible.

"And look! I have given you the seed-bearing plants throughout the earth, and all the fruit trees for your food."
— Genesis 1: 29

"The carotenoids, as well as the vitamins, minerals, and fiber that are abundant in the plant-based diet appear to play important roles in the prevention of several cancers, coronary heart disease, neural tube defects, and cataracts."
— Walter C. Willett, M. D.
Harvard School of Public Health

My personal mission is to love, care, share, and to help others understand what quality living is all about.

— Dr. Tony O'Donnell

Naturopathic Doctor

"Few people today mean what they say. Dr. Tony not only means what he says, but he walks his talk. He listens to people, cares for them and he would give them his last penny if they needed it. Dr. Tony is a true humanitarian! I feel blessed to work with him and to know him.

"He is an inspiration!"

— Maggie Hofberg, Editor

Note To Readers

This publication is designed to provide accurate and educational information regarding the subject matter covered. It is published with the understanding that neither the publisher nor the author of this book is a physician, and the ideas, procedures, and suggestions in this book are not intended as a substitute for the medical advice of a trained health professional. All matters regarding your health require medical supervision. Consult your physician before beginning any exercise/diet regime or before adopting the suggestions in this book.

In addition, the statements made by the author regarding certain products and services represent the opinions of the author alone and do not constitute a recommendation or endorsement of any product or service by the publisher. The author and publisher disclaim any liability arising directly or indirectly from the use of information in this book, or of any products herein.

Contents

Miracle SUPER FOODS That Heal

Acknowledgments

As I reflect on my life, I think of all the blessings God has given me. I'm writing the final chapter of this book in beautiful Santa Barbara, California, overlooking the Pacific Ocean. I feel so at peace, yet so happy that I could spend this time with you.

It's almost 5:20 p.m. on Sunday, December 6, 1998. The sun has already vanished for the day. I breathe the fresh air of the Pacific and I smile knowing that in some small way I have made a contribution to this wonderful world of ours. I hope you enjoy this book as much as I enjoyed writing it.

Many thanks to all who have touched my life, especially my best friend and business partner, Dan Kondos; to George, Carol, Alex and Christina Kondos, my extended family; to Anuradha Sarkar, a true Indian princess; and to composer Chris Page.

Also to Lena and Cassandra, your love and friendship inspire me. To Olivia Tracey (Miss Ireland), you are a true friend. To Gerry Peyton, Irish soccer star, thank you for your inspiration. To Gabriel Byrne, you inspired me to write and I thank you.

To Dr. Earl Mindell, thanks for your friendship. You inspire us all. To Deb and Alex Cadoux, M. D., blessings always. To Tony Robbins, who helped me take action, thank you. To Jack *Chicken Soup for the Soul*® Canfield, bless you. And to Mark Victor Hansen, who dared me to be a winner. Thank you.

To Patricia Gauthier, our friendship is a blessing. To Chris Williams, my great Irish friend. To all my teachers at college back in Ireland.

To Naomi Thomas, you are a breath of fresh air, I love you. To Shane Finnerty, thanks for being a loyal friend. To God, who inspires me every day. To all at Emerald Greens. You make my life such a joy. To Mom and Dad who showered me with love. To all my wonderful brothers and sisters, I love you deeply. To Jill, who passed away much too soon. You are deeply missed.

Miracle SUPER FOODS That Heal

Foreword

by
Mark A. Cymerint, D. C., QME, CCST

The millennium is here! At no time in our history have lay people been so assertive in questioning their doctors' prescriptions. Today, people want to live longer and to look and feel better entering their more mature years. This is why Baby Boomers and Generation Xers from two different generations thirty years apart are both searching for answers to the puzzle of health.

I'm a big believer in proper nutrition because of my education and training. For almost a decade, I have been interested in green powdered Super Foods. Several years ago, I was introduced by Dr. Tony O'Donnell to absolutely the best product on the market, Emerald Greens. It has a combination of all-natural, high-quality, whole-food supplements which cannot be matched by imitators.

As we continue to search for optimum health, we must start by reading and understanding Dr. O'Donnell's book, *Miracle Super Foods That Heal.* Its message is clear. We must change our diets, life-styles, and chemical dependencies. We must choose our supplements carefully and seek alternatives to drugs and surgery. Physical fitness is hard work, but it can be achieved. Be a leader of your life and your family's life and take responsibility for your own health.

Dr. Tony O'Donnell is an innovative front runner among nutritional leaders. His book will challenge many of the ideas you have about alternative medicines. *Miracle Super Foods That Heal* will give you a head start on getting your system up to speed with an all-in-one approach to good nutrition. This book is a winner!

Dr. Mark A. Cymerint is an international lecturer on chiropractic continuing education and nutrition, is host of the hit TV show, "Just for the Health of It," and has a chiropractic practice in Mission Viejo, California.

Take care of one another and may you have a life filled with abundant love, joy, and health. As the Irish blessing says:

> "May the road rise to meet you, may the wind be always at your back, may the sun shine warmly upon your face, the rain fall softly on your field and until we meet again may God hold you safely in the palm of his hand. Remember only one life that soon has passed, only what's done with love will last."

Blessings,

Dr. Tony O'Donnell, N.D.
Santa Barbara, California

CHAPTER ONE

Discovering My Life's Work

*"Whoever sows sparingly will also reap
sparingly, and whoever sows generously will
also reap generously."*
— II Corinthians 9:6

It was a cold, overcast day on November 12, 1979, when the phone rang. At the time I was living in Galway, Ireland. I picked up the phone and my cousin told me the sad news.

"Your father just died. He suffered a heart attack."

Daddy was the kind of man who I thought would always be with me. I had come to believe that fathers don't die. I was twenty-one at the time, working as a disc jockey waiting for that elusive big break.

Growing up in a family of eleven was not easy. I had to compete for Mom's attention with six beautiful sisters and four loving, but incredibly stubborn, brothers. I was the youngest boy, so I was spoiled. My brothers and sisters called me "Mom's Pet," or teased that I never did anything around the house.

There was not a lot of money, so we had to do the best we could. Summer holidays would be spent on the farm making hay for the local farmer. In the winter months, we found ourselves picking potatoes on cold, frosty mornings. It was tough work and our backs ached, but we were for hire and the money was decent.

We always started early in the morning around 7:30 a.m. Break time was at 10 o'clock, a welcome moment. We got hot tea delivered in a flask with lovely Irish soda bread or sometimes white bread with raspberry jam.

My father, Joe, was a very tall, strong, and proud man. Honesty and integrity meant everything to him. To bring disrespect to the family

1

meant he would give any of us an automatic flogging.

My mother is a deeply religious woman who goes to mass and prays every day. I tease her that she has "more candles and prayer books than all the people who have visited the Vatican in the past twenty-five years." She is small and plump with beautiful skin and a radiant smile. Her name is Margaret, but she likes people to call her "Mrs. O'Donnell." I always felt that she is the best mother anyone could have. She has the most gentle heart and loving manner.

When we were kids, we were always sick and going to the doctor, something I dreaded terribly. I was embarrassed to be seen as a weakling by my friends. Health and nutrition were foreign words to me. Most of our food was bacon, eggs, and sausage. That kind of a meal is now referred to as "cholesterol on a plate." But we did not know better.

Growing up, we followed what our parents did, as so many other generations had before us. We were told those foods were "good for you." It's no wonder that heart disease is rampant in Ireland and other parts of the world.

Education was important to our family, so I had a chance to go to college and earned good grades. But it was not until I turned twenty-one that my life took a big change after I received the terrible phone call that my father had died. His heart attack made me look more carefully at my own life and what I was putting into my body. It was then that I decided to dedicate my life to helping people make better choices about what to eat and what to avoid.

My personal mission is to love, care, share, and to help others understand what quality living is all about.

CHAPTER TWO

The Wonders of the Body

It's ironic that it takes something drastic like a death in the family for us to make changes in our life. I studied every book and took every course I could find on holistic healing. It has been a long, hard struggle, but I believe the benefits far outweigh the long, arduous nights I stayed at home studying books. Mom would say the rosary at bedtime. Looking back, I appreciate what she taught me. She said, "Find the love in everything you do. It is there you will find the happiness."

My happiness is healing the sick. It is a true mission of love. I believe that is what God wants me to do. So, my calling is to understand herbs and be a naturopathic doctor.

My relationship with plants began early. My father was a great gardener and he would teach me how to plant flowers, scallions, and potatoes. As a little boy, I was fascinated when seeds I put into the ground sprouted.

Thomas Edison said that until man can duplicate a blade of grass, Nature can laugh at his so-called scientific discoveries. Hippocrates told us, "Let thy food be thy medicine and thy medicine be thy food."

When I was doing research for this book, I came across some startling facts that I want to share with you. These facts are not meant to scare you, but you should be aware of them.

Cancer and heart disease are at an all time high. One in three Americans will get cancer. One million people suffer from heart disease annually. We spend roughly $1.2 trillion each year on health care. Yet, where are we? We have as much sickness today as any other time in history. I think it's time we accepted responsibility and took our health back.

Daily we are being poisoned by billions of pounds of toxic waste that are discharged into our nation's air, water, and soil. United States manufacturing facilities dump two hundred billion pounds of toxins into our air each year. Slowly, we are destroying Mother Earth. Why do we knowingly and willingly destroy the gifts God has bestowed upon this planet and humanity?

In the last two years, the Environmental Protection Agency has issued health advisories to warn about 2,000 substances that can potentially pollute waters in various parts of the nation. Further, EPA reports that 43% of water in the United States does violate federal health regulations. This affects roughly half of the population. Since the 2000 census, that's about 150 million people who are drinking water that has pollutants such as fecal matter, parasites, pesticides, lead, radiation, toxic chemicals, and disease-causing microbes.

Poisons abound in modern America. CBS News reported that 25,000 miles of U. S. waterways are contaminated. The weekly magazine *U.S. News and World Report* cited research that estimates one in six Americans drink water that has too much lead. Lead dinner plates killed the ancient Roman aristocracy. Today, its ingestion is linked to brain damage, especially in growing children.

Other poisons are the vast quantities of pesticides released into the air each year. Seventy-one percent of them are known to cause cancer in lab studies.

A hundred thousand people die from bad reactions to prescription drugs, and medical malpractice is blamed for another 100,000 deaths per year.

The stress of toxins in our brains and bodies is taking its toll in U. S. schools. At the beginning of the 21st Century, it's estimated that roughly 22 million children will be taking a prescription medicine, Ritalin, for attention deficit disorders that interfere with learning.

I could go on and on, but I will spare you the misery of sad statistics. So, what can we do? And how do we take charge and change the deteriorating world?

It begins with education. People are beginning to investigate new alternative ways to heal. The cover of *Time* magazine in a November 1998 issue asked the question: "Herbal supplements - what are they and do they work?" I think the answer is a resounding yes, but some medical professionals disagree.

However, it seems there was a huge paradigm shift in the last five years of the 20th Century towards alternative medicines. Allopathic healers who use homeopathic remedies found themselves trying to answer an increasing number of patients' questions about holistic healing.

Searching for cures beyond the American Medical Association is not always easy. There is still resistance because alternatives are not considered politically acceptable. But even some traditional medical doctors are going beyond standard prescriptions and see-you-later attitudes to seek a more holistic approach to natural healing. Similarly, there has been a huge struggle between the M.D.s and the D.C.s (Doctors of Chiropractic). Even N.D.s (Naturopathic Doctors) occasionally find themselves in hot water with their colleagues. I believe there is room for all of us who try to help patients find what works best for them.

Balance is the key. Respect is also important. If you don't like how you are treated, make changes and find what works for you. Personally, chiropractic treatment has worked very powerfully for me.

Fortunately, I've found some good medical doctors who are open-minded and who are willing to explore the uncharted territory that once seemed alien to them. For your convenience, I will recommend a partial list of books and some top U. S. health practitioners at the end of this book.

I believe that the doctors of today are becoming the nutritionists of tomorrow. Sooner or later, the healing power of herbs will come to light and prevent our loved ones from premature and untimely death.

From the Bible, God tells us that, "Behold I have given you every herb bearing seed which is upon the face of all the earth. And every tree in which is the fruit of a tree, and to every beast of the earth, and to every fowl of the air, and to everything that creepeth upon the earth, wherein there is life. I have given every green herb for meat; and it was so. And the Father of love saw everything that he had made and behold, it was very good."

I believe this passage says it all. Unfortunately, we refuse to live by the principles laid out in the Bible. The consequence is ill health in mind, body, and spirit. The good news is that sickness is preventable. In order for us to fully understand the human body, it is important that we take a look at its complex machinery.

The Human Body

The human body is a work of genius. It is so complex and so magnificent that scientists marvel at its incredible power.

- 22,000,000 tiny vessels called lacteals move lymph and emulsified fat from the intestine in digestion.
- 262 bones hold the body's soft tissues up.
- 600 muscles allow us to move.
- 970 miles of blood vessels carry about six quarts of blood that complete a lap from and to the heart every two minutes.
- 70 times a minute is the average beat of an adult human heart; 4200 times an hour, 36,792,000 times a year.
- 4 ounces of blood are expelled with each beat; 16 pounds of blood a minute; 12 tons a day; 4300 tons a year; 260,000 tons in sixty years.
- 320 cubic inches is the average adult's lung capacity; 6,000,000,000 air cells take in about 2,400 ounces of air a day through 20,000 square inches of tissue. That's equivalent to a floor 12 feet square breathing for each of us.
- 3 pounds, 2 ounces is the typical weight of a man's brain, while a woman's weighs more — 3 pounds, 12 ounces.
- 10,000,000 nerve endings connect the brain to the body.
- 40 miles of 3,500 sweat tubes run through every square inch of human skin.
- 6,000 different odors can be distinguished by the human nose.
- 20,000 hairs in human ears tune immediately to a wide range of frequencies.
- 40 pounds of pressure can be exerted by the human jaw.
- 4,000 cells on tongues allow tasting that can distinguish between fresh and foul, sweet and sour, bitter and salty, and send those signals instantly to the brain.

Miracle SUPER FOODS That Heal

A typical human is made of:
561 cubic feet hydrogen
112 cubic feet oxygen
60 cubic feet nitrogen
24 pounds carbon
10 gallons water
7 pounds lime
2 pounds phosphorous
2 ounces salt
1/4 ounce iron
1/10 pound iodine

Cost of materials? A few dollars.

In order for our bodies to function properly, we must feed them the correct foods and water. The biggest challenge we face is how to get the proper nutrients from what we eat. Crops are being sprayed with pesticides, herbicides, and insecticides. Soils become depleted of essential minerals necessary to keep body cells in good health. So, it is vitally important to supplement our diet with the correct nutrients. Since the land is often leached of minerals and we continue to spray our fruits and vegetables, what chance do we have for healthy survival? It's no wonder that people are coming down with illnesses all across the country. Scientists report that the chief causes of cancer are toxic pollutants in the environment.

We humans are destroying the earth's balance and diversity of life forms. Several companies are now marketing oxygen therapy equipment. Oxygenated water, even oxygen bars, have sprung up across the United States. I sadly predict that a day may come when we will all be required to carry oxygen tanks on our backs or in our cars. Why can't we see that ultimately we are destroying our own human future?

Where are we to go from here? What future do our children have? Luckily, there are steps we can take to ward off the onslaught of pollution and poisons.

CHAPTER THREE

How To Prevent Cancer

I dedicate this chapter to Jill Flanter, a cancer patient, who passed away much too soon. Jill was a beautiful lady whom I loved dearly. I hope that the words contained in this book will be of value in saving someone from the atrocities of cancer that took Jill's precious young life.

Cancer is multi-factorial, meaning that a lot of different factors may provoke the disease. However, experts do agree that cancer is caused by the failure of the cells to undergo normal regulated growth. Cancer researchers tell us that initial DNA damage develops into active cancer over a period of time due to DNA defects in specific target cells.

Free Radicals and Antioxidants

There is a lot of talk these days about free radicals and the damage they can cause to cells if left unchecked. But what are free radicals? Simply put, a free radical is the term for an unstable atom or group of atoms. An atom becomes unstable when it loses an electron, which often happens in cooking fats and oils through exposure to radiation and pollutants. Unpaired electrons tend to bond with other atoms to regain their stability. This changes the makeup of each of the chemicals involved in the reaction and is called oxidation. Sometimes, this causes chain reactions within the body that can lead to serious cell damage. When the damage occurs to our DNA and the DNA replicates itself, the genetic damage is copied through each subsequent replication, which perpetuates the damaged DNA. This is how free radicals get linked to cancer, the cells that go bad because their programming code is disrupted.

There are many ways in which free radicals are generated. Biochemical processes themselves naturally lead to their formation. For instance, when cells utilize oxygen to generate energy, unstable oxygen molecules are released. Diets high in fat increase free-radical activity because oxidation occurs more readily in the processing of fat molecules than it does in processing protein or carbohydrate molecules. Radiation from the sun, cigarette smoke, and car exhaust can generate free radicals.

Under normal circumstances, the body can keep free radicals in check. When excessive free-radical formation occurs, however, cell and tissue damage can occur.

This is where antioxidants come in. They safely bind to the free electrons and thus prevent any chemical damage from occurring. Common antioxidants include vitamins A, C, and E, the mineral selenium, and enzymes such as superoxide dismutase and glutathione peroxidase.

Remember that our bodies are under constant free-radical attack. If the initial DNA damage has not been repaired before a cell divides, the damage unfortunately becomes permanent due to DNA replication. Sometimes the damage is even magnified in further DNA generations. It's important to understand that free-radical hits might have happened many years before cancerous cells emerge into full blown disease.

If antioxidant levels are low, the danger of getting cancer or other debilitating diseases is high. Fortunately, green foods are tremendous cancer fighters. They are loaded with phytonutrients that block or eliminate free radicals. The Emerald Greens product is extremely rich in antioxidants.

A recent Framingham, Massachusetts study indicates that five to seven servings of green leafy vegetables will reduce cancer by sixty-six percent. Yet, most Americans do not eat enough vegetables.

I highly suggest that you take care and accept full responsibility for your health from this moment forward.

Emerald Greens has all of the do's. But since we live in such a toxic world, it is necessary to take even more supplements such as vegicaps or powders for full absorption and heed the following don'ts.

Don'ts

- Don't eat highly processed foods or foods containing chemical preservatives or artificial coloring.
- Don't eat commercial meat that has stilbestrol (DES), antibiotics or other chemicals.
- Don't eat fried foods and don't use heat-treated oils with preservatives or hydrogenated shortening.
- Don't eat canned fruits or vegetables. Most of these are over-sweetened and many vegetables are over-cooked.
- Don't smoke! Give up cigarettes completely.
- Don't drink much alcohol.
- Don't drink coffee.
- Don't eat much fat.
- Don't hold onto the past with resentment, anger, or fear.

Do's

- Aim for the following calorie distribution each day:
  30% in proteins
  20% in fats
  50% unrefined carbohydrates
- Eat lots of fresh fruits.
- Eat lots of fresh vegetables.
- Drink lots of green tea.
- Take grape-seed extract.
- Take vitamins A, B, C, and E.
- Walk, jog, or run every other day.
- Have regular medical check-ups.
- Reduce stress as much as possible.
- Love as much as possible and let go of anger and fear.
- Forgive those who have hurt you, because resentment is toxic.
- Smile often.
- Go see a good movie.
- Laugh out loud. Smiling, relaxing, and laughing all release endorphins that make you feel good.
- Light a candle and close your eyes. Say some special prayers or meditate.

Miracle SUPER FOODS That Heal

- Say the following: "I release and let go of any discomfort I feel in my body from this moment forward." Say it five times. Then before you open your eyes, say firmly, "I embrace love and abundant health from this moment forward."

Nutritional Quantity Terms

1 gram (g) = 1/1000 kilogram (kg), or 1000 milligrams (mg)

1 milligram (mg) = 1/1000 gram (g), or 1000 micrograms (mcg)

1 microgram (mcg) = 1/1,000,000 (g)

1 Retinol Equivalent (RE) = Unit measure for Vitamin

3.3 International Unit (IU) = 1 RE if source is animal;
   or 10 IU = 1 RE if source is plant beta-carotene

CHAPTER FOUR

Super Foods,
Acerola to Wheat Sprouts

*"The earth is the Lord's and the fullness thereof, the world
and those who dwell therein, for he has founded it upon the seas
and established it upon the rivers."*

- Psalm 24:1-2

After years of study, research, and poring over hundreds of books, I formulated a product that has made a difference in the lives of thousands of people. The product is called Emerald Greens Herbal Super Food. This is not just another product so that I or someone else can make a profit. Emerald Greens is a gift from God. The testimonials I receive are so rewarding that I want to share some at the end of this book.

I was motivated to develop Emerald Greens for my mother after my dad died. I realized back then that I did not know much about herbs and proper nutrition. But I knew my father was a heavy smoker and had suffered a heart attack. Then he went to the local hospital for a flu shot. A young intern gave the injection on a Friday and Dad died that Sunday. Our family doctor said later he should never have had a flu shot following the heart attack. Accidents do happen, but I think it was the intern's inexperience and a sloppy hospital policy that killed my father.

There are about 3,400 heart attacks every day in the United States. That translates into $3.5 billion a year for the medical industry. Recent research tells us that most heart attacks happen on a Monday morning as people go to stressful jobs that are not fulfilling for the mind, body, or soul.

I created Emerald Greens to really make a difference in my mother's and other people's lives. It is a remarkable combination of super foods with thirty health-boosting ingredients.

Super foods generally are organically grown in a chemical-free environment. The foods are dried for preservation with air, not heat, in order to preserve enzymes. It's my conviction that anything heated over 100 degrees Fahrenheit loses its therapeutic healing properties.

These concentrated super foods are a potent source of vitamins, minerals, enzymes, antioxidants, fiber, and essential amino acids, which reputedly add alkalinity to our system, balance us, increase our energy, improve stamina, sharpen mental acuity, and deodorize and cleanse the cells and colon.

Emerald Greens is for people who want to get their nutrients and minerals from a whole food versus a vitamin tablet. It's important to remember that it's not the number of vitamins you take, but their form. Always buy capsules instead of tablets. Capsules are digested and absorbed better in the body. See Glossary for details about vitamins and minerals.

Emerald Greens is a powder with living enzymes that break down nutrients as soon as they enter the body. These highly concentrated food powders filled with nutrients can be mixed with water, juice, or blendered ice for a delicious smoothie or drink.

There are no fillers or binders in Emerald Greens. There is no MSG, no coloring dyes, no kelp, no alcohol, no preservatives, no added salts, starches, maltodextrin, gluten, corn, fats, oil stabilizers, casein, or milk derivatives.

Although I always recommend consulting with a physician prior to starting a new nutritional program, I feel that this product is so pure that even a child can take it. Many mothers do have their children on Emerald Greens and write to tell me how their children's health seems greatly improved.

The impact of Emerald Greens is truly amazing. I have never seen a product deliver the incredible results that this powdered formula does. People constantly tell me they feel better soon after consumption.

The following super foods are in every serving of Emerald Greens.

Miracle SUPER FOODS That Heal

1. Acerola Berry Juice Powder
Caribbean Cherry or Berry

100 Milligrams (Mg)
in one serving (3 teaspoons) of Emerald Greens

Fact:
Most vitamin C pills and supplements labeled
"natural" are made from acerola.

Since the body does not store vitamin C, it must be replenished on a daily basis. Without question, the bright red acerola berry is one of the most potent natural sources of vitamin C anywhere, containing sixteen to eighteen percent highly absorbable ascorbic acid. Most vitamin C pill supplements labeled "natural" are made from acerola.

For Emerald Greens, the berries are first juiced. The juice is then spray-dried into powder which provides 100 mg of vitamin C per serving. Vitamin C helps elevate levels of high-density lipoproteins (HDLs), the so-called good cholesterol, which protects the heart and reduces the risk of heart attacks.

The late Nobel Prize laureate, Linus Pauling, praised the medical benefits of vitamin C. He showed that it is both antiviral and antibacterial and strengthens the immune system.

Vitamin C has been used successfully to treat a long list of illnesses ranging from ulcers, scurvy, and arthritis to cancer, high blood pressure, eye problems, and the common cold.

According to James E. Enstrom, M.D., at the University of California, people who consume 300 to 400 milligrams (mgs) of vitamin C on a daily basis lengthened their average life expectancy by six years. Dr. Enstrom also studied women who consumed a few hundred milligrams of vitamin C daily. Their death rate from heart disease and cancer was reduced by ten percent, equivalent to one extra year of life.

How much vitamin C should you take? Dr. Pauling, who lived to be nearly 100, thought several grams a day would help everyone. More traditional recommended daily doses are 500 to 1,000 milligrams. My mentor, Jay Patrick, was also a friend of Linus Pauling. Jay takes about 20 grams of vitamin C a day. I personally take 4,000 to 8,000 milligrams each day.

Acerola berry juice is also a rich source of antioxidants, which help fight aging. Acerola enhances the absorption of a bioflavonoid called quercitin and helps balance the pH in the colon.

2. Alfalfa Juice Powder (organic)
Alfalfa Leaves

430 Milligrams (Mg)
in one serving (3 teaspoons) of Emerald Greens

Fact:
Alfalfa grows a root system ten to twenty feet deep, which draws many raw nutrients from soil such as potassium, phosphorus, iron, calcium, vitamins A and C.

Alfalfa is a lentil, not a grass, and is one of the most nourishing green plants on earth. Alfalfa roots gather minerals from ten to twenty feet down, growing deeper into soil than most any other vegetables.

Ten grams of alfalfa has 8,000 IUs of beta-carotene and 200,000 IUs of vitamin K, which helps blood clot properly. Alfalfa also has healthy quantities of vitamins D and E and minerals such as phosphorus, potassium, magnesium, and calcium.

In addition, this super food contains betaine, a substance that combines with hydrochloride in the stomach to form hydrochloric acid, which is necessary to easily break down food.

The chlorophyll in alfalfa, as in all green plants, helps to deodorize the intestinal tract and to detoxify the liver, lungs, and colon. Chlorophyll inhibits the growth and development of unfriendly bacteria and might interfere with the protein digestive enzymes in cancer cells. Moreover, chlorophyll is excellent as a blood builder and blood rejuvenator.

The chlorophyll molecule contains a ring structure that is identical to the rings found in the hemoglobin molecule—except for one difference. The center of the chlorophyll molecule has a magnesium atom. The center of the hemoglobin molecule has an iron atom. It's fair to say, as the poet Dylan once wrote, "the force that fuses through the green stem fuses through me." Blood and chlorophyll are so similar, yet chlorophyll can help cleanse toxins from blood.

3. Apple Pectin and Fiber
Whole Apple

670 Milligrams (Mg)
in one serving (3 teaspoons) of Emerald Greens

Fact:
The water-soluble complex carbohydrate and fiber in apples bind bile acids and withdraw cholesterol from blood, which helps reduce risk of heart disease; also lower or stabilize blood sugar levels.

Apple pectin and apple fiber help intestines sustain rhythmic contractions necessary for regular elimination. Most people have poor elimination because the bowel is one of the most neglected and ignored parts of a person's body. Daily, we fill up with all the wrong foods. The typical western diet contains food that takes between seventy-five and one hundred hours to go from the mouth to the toilet. Parasites, germs, and worms accumulate on the walls of the colon as fecal matter builds up.

The average person carries anywhere from seven to twenty-five pounds of dried fecal matter stuck in the colon. Even in small quantities, poisons from a toxic colon can harm the body. Some medical doctors think that ninety-five percent of all illness begins in the colon. Every year in the United States, two million men and women are diagnosed with colon cancer; forty-four percent of them die.

According to Dr. Bernard Jenson, nutritionist and author, "Every tissue in the body is fed by the bloodstream, which is supplied by the bowel. When the bowel is dirty, the blood is also dirty and so are the organs and tissues. ...The bowel must be cared for first before any effective healing can take place."

Excessive use of laxatives can be hazardous to your health, too. It is far safer to cleanse the body naturally through diet. For years, the Chinese have used nutritional combinations to promote the essential bodily functions that we associate with good health such as cleansing the intestines.

After studying these Chinese methods, I find it absolutely necessary to include their dietary ingredients in the Emerald Greens formula. So,

Emerald Greens contains colon cleansers that work in harmony with the body to balance organs and glands: apple pectin and fiber, brown rice, and sprouted barley malt.

One of the most important cleansers is apple pectin and fiber for regular bowel movements. These fibers cleanse the colon walls and at the same time allow liposomes to form, which help nutrients to be properly absorbed into the blood stream. In the blood, apple pectin and fiber also help to eliminate cholesterol and inhibit the absorption of heavy metals and toxins that come our way in the air we breathe, the food we eat, and the water we drink.

Emerald Greens contains a plentiful supply of fiber to ensure proper elimination. As any mother will tell you, a tiny baby will eat and eliminate. Poor diet, over-consumption of food, lack of water and exercise, stress, late night binging, and taking antibiotics can cause a sluggish, unhealthy digestive tract.

Take care of your colon. Choose carefully what you put into your body. You have only one.

4. Astragalus Root (Milk Vetch)
Astragalus membranaceus
Chinese call it *huang chi*

80 Milligrams (Mg)
in one serving (3 teaspoons) of Emerald Greens

Fact:
Chinese physicians prescribe astragalus as an immune booster for cancer patients after chemotherapy or radiation.

Of all the herbs that enhance our immune system, astragalus — or milk vetch root — is perhaps the most effective. Astragalus is one of the largest groups of flowering plants with roughly 1,750 documented species. Some of its forms such as locoweed are highly toxic. But the astragalus found in health food stores is safe to eat.

The species used for medical treatment is commonly found in China and grows abundantly in open woods or along the edges of forests. Astragalus can be ingested in many forms including tea, tinctures, capsules, powders, and its dried root. The roots are usually harvested after a particular plant is four or five years old. The roots are sliced into pieces that look like tongue depressors. Those pieces are then generally boiled in an herb cooker and the juice bottled and refrigerated. Astragalus is good for you, either hot or cold.

This root is the most widely used herb in China, where it has been prescribed as a medical treatment for at least two thousand years. In traditional Chinese medicine, astragalus is used as an immune-enhancing tonic for the treatment of fatigue, loss of appetite, diarrhea, cancer, and blood disorders. The root can also be used in combination with other herbs to help restore what the Chinese call Qi (pronounced "chee"), the energy of life.

Astragalus is an adaptogenic herb which means it helps restore balance and normal functioning to a disrupted body system. Herbalists think that astragalus enhances the immune system and promotes tissue regeneration through substances called polysaccharides which astragalus root has in abundance.

Miracle SUPER FOODS That Heal

Scientific studies of the root in the 1970s confirmed the plant's ability to stimulate the human immune system, which helps the body to fight viruses and bacteria. The research data showed that astragalus was able to *quadruple* the ability of body cells to fight off disease.

Astragalus has also been used successfully to treat patients who have undergone chemotherapy. As many of us know, chemotherapy and radiation have a tendency to suppress the immune system and make a patient vulnerable to other opportunistic diseases.

In 1975, researchers began a study that showed how astragalus supplements enhanced bone marrow production of white blood cells, the body's first line of defense against foreign microorganisms such as bacteria and viruses. The researchers also documented that astragalus neutralized toxins in patients undergoing chemotherapy and radiation treatments. After taking astragalus, their quality of life increased positively. Some researchers also think that astragalus increases sperm mobility, which can help with infertility problems.

In the United States, astragalus is mainly used to treat colds, flu, and chronic fatigue and as an overall strengthening and conditioning elixir. Astragalus has many other adaptogenic capabilities such as helping to reduce blood pressure, dilate blood vessels, improve blood circulation, and protect the liver from toxicities.

Astragalus is safe to use, but there is a caution with all herbs if you are pregnant, breast feeding or have any serious medical conditions. In those cases, please check with your nutritionist, doctor, or other healthcare practitioner before ingesting.

Miracle SUPER FOODS That Heal

5. Barley Grass Leaf Juice Powder (Organic)
Barley Leaves

430 Milligrams (Mg)
in one serving (3 teaspoons) of Emerald Greens

Fact:
Barley has lignan phytochemicals (antioxidants), which
bind with free radicals and help prevent cell damage.

Barley is a cereal grass that has been cultivated for food for thousands of years. In its young, growing "green stage," researchers know that it has many times the level of vitamins, minerals, enzymes, and proteins found in mature cereal plants.

Researcher Dr. Yoshihide Hagiwara thinks that green barley is the "ideal fast food" because juice in the young barley leaves contains potassium, calcium, magnesium, organic iron, copper, phosphorus, manganese, zinc, chlorophyll, and the enzyme superoxide dismutase (SOD).

Barley juice powder contains four times more vitamin B than whole wheat flour and thirty times more than milk. Barley contains three times more vitamin C than spinach and seven times more than oranges. It even contains five times more iron than liver.

Howard Lutz, M.D., Director, Institute of Preventative Medicine in Washington, D. C. says, "Barley grass improves stamina and clarity of thought, and reduces addiction to things that are bad for you. It improves the texture of the skin and heals the dryness associated with aging."

Research by Professor Takayuki Shibamoto, Chairman of the Environmental Toxicology Division at the University of California-Davis, is studying an antioxidant compound in young green barley that he says is as potent as beta-carotene, vitamin C, or vitamin E.

Barley grass extract can reduce inflammation and contains enzymes that can inactivate and break down carcinogens such as tobacco tar. Barley's high fiber content helps the colon to move properly and helps eliminate toxin build-ups that can cause disease. That is why barley grass is associated with energy boosts, lowering cholesterol, and even helping people who suffer the pains of arthritis.

6. Bee Pollen
Natural pollen from flowers.

250 Milligrams (Mg)
in one serving (3 teaspoons) of Emerald Greens

Fact:
Pollen is the yellow, powderlike male sex cells on flower stamens gathered by bees to provide the essential proteins necessary to rear young bees.

For centuries, various cultures have used bee pollen for medical treatment. The pollen is gathered by a device placed at the hive's entrance so that the pollen on bee legs brushes off as the flying insects move in and out.

Undisturbed in the hive, bee pollen contains up to thirty percent moisture. That is why pollen will turn rancid and become contaminated by mold and mildew if not quickly frozen. Therefore, it is imperative that bee pollen be dried carefully to preserve its potency and nutritional value.

Bee pollen has been described by many as Nature's most perfect food. Twenty-five percent of its weight is a protein that contains eighteen amino acids. Its other ingredients are impressive: a dozen vitamins including A, B-complex, C, D, E; twenty-eight minerals; fatty acids; carbohydrates; and eleven enzymes or co-enzymes. Bee pollen also contains high amounts of superoxide dismutase, lecithin, beta-carotene, and selenium. All of these elements help the gastrointestinal system to absorb nutrients.

Many allergy sufferers have found relief by ingesting bee pollen as a natural antihistamine. The pollen stimulates the immune system as well, and has been found helpful to overcome nausea, sleep disorders, and urinary and rectal problems after radiation treatments. Bee pollen might also help relieve anemia, cerebral hemorrhage, colitis, and constipation.

7. Beet Juice Powder
Root

250 Milligrams
in one serving (3 teaspoons) of Emerald Greens

Fact:
Beets have significant concentrations of carotenoids and flavonoids which work as antioxidants, reduce accumulation of plaque in arteries, promote cell differentiation and resist cancer, cleanse blood, and help circulation.

The beet vegetable is a red root whose green stems and leaves are also edible. Beets are so naturally sweet that commercial sweeteners are produced from them.

Beets were used in ancient times to help gastrointestinal disorders and pain. Modern researchers have been able to identify large concentrations of carotenoids and flavonoids in beets. There are more than 600 carotenoids so far identified. In addition to the red pigment in beets, many are the bright yellow and orange pigments in sweet potatoes, winter squash, carrots, apricots, and papayas. The best known is beta-carotene concentrated in carrots, which the body converts to vitamin A.

Carotenoids are powerful antioxidants and boost cancer resistance. Some carotenoids also help protect against cardiovascular disease and macular degeneration in eyes.

8. Bilberry
Vaccinium myrtillus
Wild blueberries smaller than commercial blueberries.
Berries Extract

10 Milligrams (Mg)
in one serving (3 teaspoons) of Emerald Greens

Fact:
Bilberry contains compounds called anthocyanosides,
natural antioxidants that protect small blood vessels
(capillaries) from free radical damage and improve
circulation and eyesight.

Bilberry became very popular during World War II when Royal Air
Force pilots in England reported better night vision when they ate bilberry jam. The European bilberry is composed of twenty-five percent
anthrocyanandin pigments, which are necessary for healthy vision.
Bilberry also improves blood circulation in the eye retina and regenerates
retinal purple, a substance needed for good eyesight.

In the 1960s, French scientists documented that enzyme action in
the eye was enhanced after bilberry was eaten. Recent research shows that
bilberry extracts markedly improve eye adaptation to darkness, which is
the amount of time it takes for eyes to adjust to dark after exposure to
light, artificial or sunlight. Bilberry has even helped people with myopia,
in which long-distance images are blurred. I have seen remarkable results
in people who use bilberry. One registered pharmacist in Las Vegas wrote
to tell me that she no longer needs her glasses.

Bilberry flavonoid extract has been shown in medical studies to
strengthen capillary walls, which helps prevent transient ischemic strokes
caused by blood leaks if the capillary tissue is weak. Bilberry also strengthens larger blood vessel walls and inhibits blood platelet aggregation,
which helps prevent both hemorrhaging and blood clots. Bilberry's ability to strengthen blood vessels was shown in an experiment with patients
who suffered hypertension from stress. Bilberry flavonoids helped to prevent permeability and blood leakage in their brain capillaries.

Miracle SUPER FOODS That Heal

9. Brown Rice Germ and Bran
Whole rice seeds with husk and vitamin-rich bran embryo

400 Milligrams (Mg)
in one serving (3 teaspoons) of Emerald Greens

Fact:
Rice bran contains not only vitamins and minerals, but insoluble fiber, which helps cleanse intestines and lowers blood cholesterol.

Rice is the staple food for two-thirds of the world's population. In Asia, where rice has been grown for thousands of years, rice is considered sacred food. Rice is different from most grains in that it is normally consumed in its kernel form. Rice kernels from the paddy are encased in husks that are not edible and must be removed before cooking. After shelling the husks, what remains is brown rice with bran layers that surround the kernels. These light brown layers not only give rice its color and nut-like flavor, but the bran-layer fiber is rich in vitamins and minerals.

Much of the rice sold in the United States, however, has been extensively milled to remove the outer layers of bran to produce white or "polished" rice. To market a firmer, fluffier rice, some mills parboil the kernels. In that process, the rough rice is soaked, steamed under pressure, and then dried before milling, which strips the food of most nutritional value.

Fortunately, the highly nutritious bran is retained in the Emerald Greens formula. Rice bran is an excellent source of thiamin, niacin, vitamin B-6, iron, phosphorous, magnesium, potassium, vitamin E, silicon, and a correct balance of amino acids. Unlike wheat, rice bran is non-allergenic and free of gluten.

Most importantly, brown rice germ and bran provide soluble and insoluble fibers necessary for intestinal cleansing. Brown rice helps to detoxify, deodorize, and cleanse the intestines while at the same time it helps to speed bowel transit time. Soluble fiber found in rice bran might even help lower cholesterol levels by binding to food cholesterol, which is eliminated from the digestive tract.

10. Chlorella Algae (Cracked Cell)
Chlorella pyrenoidosa
Edible, single-celled plant that lives in fresh water.

250 Milligrams (Mg)
in one serving (3 teaspoons) of Emerald Greens

Fact:
Japanese researchers report that chlorella algae can raise
the level of protein albumin in the blood. Albumin is one
of the body's most powerful antioxidants, which transports
toxins to the liver and moves vitamins, minerals, fatty acids,
hormones, and other substances throughout the body.

Chlorella is a one-celled, fresh-water algae that has been on this
earth for at least 2.5 billion years, half the age of our planet. According
to scientists, chlorella has survived in modern times because of its
inherent ability to repair its own DNA. Chlorella can multiply quickly,
quadrupling itself every seventeen to twenty hours under optimum
growing conditions.

If you are a vegetarian, it would be wise to consider adding chlorella to your diet as a good non-meat source of protein. Sixty percent of the
algae is an easily digested protein that is twice the amount in soy and
eight times the amount in rice. Beyond its high protein content, chlorella contains more than twenty vitamins and minerals, including B-1, B-2, B-
6, B-12, beta-carotene, vitamins E and K, liberal amounts of iron, zinc,
phosphorus, potassium, sulphur, cobalt, copper, iodine, calcium, magnesium, manganese, and nucleic acids, which help cells to regenerate.

By weight, this single-celled algae contains an enormous amount of
chlorophyll, twenty times the content of alfalfa, nearly ten times that of
spirulina (dried algae tablets) and eight times wheat grass. Chlorophyll
detoxifies and deodorizes the mouth, colon, blood, and cells.

Chlorella also contains 180 milligrams per 100 grams of the antioxidant, beta-carotene. When beta-carotene is combined with vitamin E in
food for cancer patients, the two powerful antioxidants work together to
block and destroy cancer cells.

The incidence of cancer in Japan is low compared to the rest of the world — only one in forty people. In contrast, one out of three people in the United States has cancer and one out of eight in Canada.

Why should Japan have such a low cancer rate? Probably it's their diet comprised mostly of fish, green tea, and chlorella. Chlorella is a common food throughout Japan where it is eaten to help protect against radiation and highly toxic air pollution. Scientific studies have confirmed that the algae helps remove pesticides and heavy metals such as cadmium and PCBs from body systems. Chlorella algae has also been shown to protect the liver from toxic overloads of poisons such as ethionine.

Japanese researchers also report that chlorella algae can raise the level of protein albumin in the blood. Albumin is one of the body's most powerful antioxidants, which transports toxins to the liver and moves vitamins, minerals, fatty acids, hormones, and other substances throughout the body. I have seen several of my patients improve dramatically after taking chlorella on a regular basis. One young man told me he stopped using drugs and alcohol once he started using chlorella.

Of all the algae's many remarkable medical benefits, the most important might be its ability to stimulate the immune system. Chlorella seems to enhance the work of macrophages, which are large cells located in many body tissues including the liver, spleen, lymph nodes, thymus, lungs, and joints. Macrophages help to eliminate harmful substances from the blood in a process known as phagocytosis.

Since increasing macrophage production can accelerate destruction of cancer cells and harmful bacteria, chlorella might be particularly beneficial for people suffering from cancer or HIV. Chlorella is also helpful for patients who have skin problems and burns. In one study, burn wounds healed twenty-five percent faster when chlorella was applied.

Chlorella is praised by many people for helping treat a wide variety of illnesses, including allergies and asthma. It also lowers cholesterol and blood pressure, reduces hardening of the arteries, and helps fight chronic fatigue.

Miracle SUPER FOODS That Heal

11. D-Alpha Tocopherol Acetate, Vitamin E
Synthetic

100 Milligrams (Mg)
in one serving (3 teaspoons) of Emerald Greens

Fact:
The May 1993 *New England Journal of Medicine* reported that 87,000 registered female nurses and 40,000 male health professionals who consumed at least 100 IU of vitamin E supplements daily for eight years had a 40% reduced risk of heart disease.

Vitamin E was first discovered in the 1920s when research showed it plays an important role in the fertility of rats. That is when vitamin E gained a reputation as a reproductive aid and was given the Greek name Tocopherol, which means "to give birth."

Since the human body does not manufacture vitamin E, it can only get into our bodies through the foods we eat. Good sources of vitamin E are vegetable oils, butter, seeds, wheat germ, whole cereal grains, nuts, egg yolks, and green leafy vegetables such as spinach and lettuce.

The recommended daily allowance for vitamin E is 30 IUs, but recent studies suggest that three times that amount, or nearly 100 IUs, is necessary for optimal health. But to ingest 100 IUs of vitamin E daily from foods would mean eating at least 11.5 ounces of almonds, or 4.5 cups of wheat germ, or about 18.5 cups of spinach. That is why vitamin E supplements are common, safe, and include non-toxic doses up to 400 to 800 IUs. Taking higher doses might cause some adverse effects.

Vitamin E is most famous for its antioxidant protection. It helps prevent skin and cell destruction from toxic elements in air, water, and food. Its main arena is the lungs, where it combines with oxygen in the blood to help maintain the proper fluidity of red blood cells that carry oxygen. Red blood cells transport life-supporting oxygen from the lungs to the capillaries which feed tissues. In that process, vitamin E reduces oxidation effects.

An illustration of this can be found in an experiment performed at the University of Texas Southwestern Medical Center. Subjects given 400 IUs of vitamin E over an eight-week period showed both a marked reduction in cholesterol levels and a decrease in free-radical oxidation.

Vitamin E also modulates abnormal blood thickening, which can cause blood clots in arteries. In a 1987 study of women who took oral contraceptives, vitamin E supplements minimized the tendency of blood platelets to stick together. That was an important finding because strokes caused by platelet aggregation are reputedly a potential and negative risk to women who take contraceptive pills.

If there is a problem with excessive bleeding, vitamin E helps control it and seems to enhance healing of wounds with less scar tissue.

Vitamin E also helps women reduce the risk of developing fibrocystic breast disease. In one study, eighty-five percent of women given vitamin E supplements responded favorably. Cysts and tenderness totally disappeared in thirty-eight percent of the patients.

Vitamin E also helps reduce painful leg and arm cramps, calms nerves, lessens pre-menstrual syndrome symptoms, reduces age or liver spots, and protects the lungs against environmental toxins.

12. Dulse of Nova Scotia
Edible Atlantic seaweed herb such as arame,
nori, kombu, hijiki, and wakame

250 Milligrams (Mg)
in one serving (3 teaspoons) of Emerald Greens

Fact:
There are more than 2,500 varieties of seaweed, which
provide a wide spectrum of minerals such as calcium,
copper, iodine, iron, magnesium, and potassium.

Dulse is a purple and red seaweed that contains generally more minerals than land plants do. As soils become depleted of natural minerals, ocean plants such as dulse will be an increasingly important supply of food. In Iceland, dulse has been used as a food for almost 2,000 years. In Ireland, dulse is harvested for mouthwash and to make seaweed soup.

In her book, *The Food Pharmacy,* Jean Carper writes, "Modern science confirms that seaweed is one of nature's all-round pharmaceutical miracles, full of chemicals that can accomplish everything from warding off and treating several types of cancer, lowering blood cholesterol and blood pressure, thinning the blood, preventing ulcers, killing bacteria and even curing constipation."

Like its cousin, kelp, dulse is a good source of iodine, which keeps the thyroid gland healthy. Moreover, dulse has one of the highest iron concentrations of any plant. It also has potassium, calcium, magnesium, boron, lithium, fluoride, and B vitamins.

Most of the dulse sold in the United States is harvested off the coast of Nova Scotia from May through August. It is picked by hand at low tide and brought to spreading grounds to dry. Dulse tastes sweet after it is dried.

These days, you can purchase dulse at most health food stores. Try it first as a condiment and add small quantities to salads and soups.

13. *Echinacea angustifolia*
(Purple Coneflower)
The Immune Booster Herb

80 Milligrams (Mg)
in one serving (3 teaspoons) of Emerald Greens

Fact:
German scientists have studied *Echinacea* and report the herb
has anti-inflammatory and immune-boosting properties.

For centuries, the North American Plains Indians used various
species of *Echinacea* to treat snake bites and illnesses. Its therapeutic value
was reportedly "discovered" by European settlers in the fall of 1885 in
Pawnee City, Nebraska. Then pioneering pharmacists such as the Lloyd
brothers of Cincinnati, Ohio developed the herbal extract.

An early researcher, Dr. J. Fearn, discovered that *Echinacea* reduced
fevers and improved circulation. He concluded that the herb provokes the
kidneys, skin, and bowels to speed up elimination of poisonous toxins.

Dr. Finley Ellingwood described *Echinacea*'s affect on saliva flow. He
claimed that the herb aided systemic secretion and excretion.

In 1937, the American Medical Association stopped research and
use of echinacea. But German and other European companies continued
to manufacture and sell it.

In 1978, Dr. P. Viehmann carried out an extensive study in
Germany. He reported a 91.5% success rate in healing wounds with a
topical *Echinacea* ointment. Since the 1980s, millions of Americans have
used the herb, especially *Echinacea purpureia*, to help fight off flu and colds.
It can be prepared in tinctures, capsules, creams, and powders. To ensure
enzymes are not damaged during harvest, the plants are always cut at the
same stage of growth.

Echinacea has been hailed as the king of blood purifiers because it
helps the macrophage "trash collectors" in blood clean up. *Echinacea* also
helps pull waste out of the lymph glands while it strengthens and conditions the lymphatic system.

The herb's most important immune-enhancing compounds are its large polysaccharides that promote T-cell growth. T-cells are strong attackers of foreign microbes in the body's immune defense system. In one German experiment, scientists discovered that polysaccharides in *Echinacea* increased T-cell activity by nearly thirty percent more than other drugs designed to trigger T-cell response.

Other studies show that *Echinacea* inhibits the formation of an enzyme that destroys natural barriers between healthy tissue and harmful organisms. What's more, *Echinacea* aids in the production of interferon, a cellular protein produced to combat viruses that infect cells. *Echinacea* might even help fight off malignant tumor cells.

The herb acts as a natural antibiotic against staph and strep infections. Its antibacterial properties are useful in healing wounds, burns, ulcers, psoriasis, acne, and eczema.

Its anti-inflammatory agents might help relieve arthritis. Other applications include treatment for snake bites, bee stings, headaches, allergies, and the common cold. A combination of *Echinacea,* goldenseal and vitamin C taken together is often recommended at the first sign of a cold or flu to blunt the viruses.

Herbalists argue about whether *Echinacea* should be taken every day. Some think it is important to give your body a break. My suggestion as a naturopathic doctor is to experiment and find the dosage that seems to work best for you.

14. *Ginkgo biloba*
Maidenhair Tree
Leaves Extract 24%

30 Milligrams (Mg)
in one serving (3 teaspoons) of Emerald Greens

Fact:
The October 1997 *Journal of the American Medical Association* published research about *Ginkgo biloba*'s ability to slow Alzheimer's disease "related to its antioxidant properties which ...act as scavengers for free radicals, considered the mediators of the excessive lipid peroxidation and cell damage observed in Alzheimer's disease."

Ginkgo biloba is related to the order Ginkgoales, which have grown on earth since the Permian period of the Paleozoic era, some 286 million to 245 million years ago. Extinct genera are known from fossilized leaves that are similar to those of the present-day tree. The ginkgo is native to China where monks revere it as a sacred herb. The word "biloba" means two lobes, like a couple of Japanese fans held together at the base. The tree is resistant to fungus and insects and can survive adverse conditions from cold to smog. But ice ages destroyed them in North America where the trees once grew abundantly.

It is a remarkable plant that is capable of repairing its own DNA. *Ginkgo biloba* first reached modern public attention in the 1950s when a German doctor named Willmar Schwabe published in scientific journals about his study of ginkgo extract produced from fifty pounds of leaves. Based on Dr. Schwabe's research, *Ginkgo biloba* became the herbal medicine of choice among doctors and pharmacists worldwide.

Ginkgo's popularity is due in part to its remarkable ability to increase blood circulation, both to the brain and to various extremities of the body. In one major study, a fifty-seven percent increase in blood flow through capillaries in toe and finger nails was documented after *Ginkgo biloba* extract was ingested. Today, doctors recommend ginkgo for the prevention and treatment of circulatory problems associated with aging.

Miracle SUPER FOODS That Heal

Further, Dr. Donald Brown studied ginkgo's affect on blood platelet aggregation, which can cause blood clots. He found that *Ginkgo biloba* inhibits platelet aggregation and also regulates the tone and elasticity of blood vessels. Moreover, ginkgo has an ability to enhance oxygen metabolism by increasing cellular uptake of glucose. The result is an energy boost.

The benefits of better blood circulation include improved memory, faster reaction time, increased energy, and improved mental acuity. *Ginkgo biloba* is also a very powerful antioxidant and research shows that it might protect the brain against free-radical damage. Furthermore, substances in ginkgo called ginkgolides have been shown to relieve allergies and asthma.

For these reasons, *Ginkgo biloba* has been used to treat a broad range of maladies including Alzheimer's disease, head injuries, cerebrovascular problems, strokes, heart attacks, poor circulation, tinnitus in the ears, vertigo, macular degeneration of the eyes, and even trauma. Ginkgo has also been successfully tried in the treatment of attention deficit disorder (A.D.D.) and multiple sclerosis.

Doses as high as 200 mg can be used in the beginning of treatment. Later, a lower maintenance dose should suffice. There are no known side effects in taking ginkgo. However, if you are pregnant or breast feeding, it is not recommended.

15. Grape-Seed Extract

10 Milligrams (Mg)
in one serving (3 teaspoons) of Emerald Greens

Fact:
Flavonoids known as proanthocyanidins are antioxidants that
are 50 times more potent than vitamin E, are concentrated in
the seeds of white and green grapes, and can help neutralize
cancer-causing free radicals found in tobacco smoke,
processed foods, and barbecued meats.

Grape-seed extract has received much press and TV exposure in the
last few years. The reason is its antioxidant properties. Research shows
grape-seed extract acts as an antioxidant fifty times more powerfully than
vitamin E and twenty times more than vitamin C. The history that lead to
the value of grape seeds goes back to the Sixteenth Century.

In 1534, the French explorer, Jacques Cartier, and his crew were
exploring the Gulf of Saint Lawrence. Trapped by an ice storm, Cartier's
men were forced to live on salted meat and biscuits. Some twenty-five
men died and another fifty became seriously ill. The problem was scurvy
caused by a vitamin C deficiency. At the time there were no cures for
scurvy. But Cartier and his men were lucky. A native North American
Indian used an old folk remedy and fed them the bark of pine trees.
Cartier wrote about the treatment in his log book, which was not read
again for four hundred years.

Then in 1966, Dr. Jacques Masquelier and his research team at the
University of Bordeaux in France discovered that what the pine bark contains is flavonoids. Those flavonoids are full of vitamin C and water-soluble proanthocyanadins (PCOs). When pine bark extract is analyzed, it
contains eighty-five percent proanthocyanadins. But grape-seed extract
has even more: ninety-five percent. The remaining five percent are the
pine cellulose and other nutrients.

In 1951, Dr. Masquelier patented his method of extracting PCOs
from pine bark and patented a second method in 1970 for extracting
PCOs from grape seeds. I have studied his work and found that he per-

sonally favored the grape-seed extract, presumably because it has the most PCO content, which is a non-toxic antioxidant.

Another argument for using grape seeds instead of pine bark is a chemical difference in processing. For pine bark, toxic chloroform must be used to extract proanthocyanadins. Consequently, many people refuse to take pine bark extract. PCOs can be extracted from grape seeds without harsh chemicals. In France, only the PCOs extracted from grape seeds are approved for medical use.

Personally, after reading scientific literature based on thirty years of clinical research, I also prefer grape-seed extract, which has the added value of Gallic esters that bind with free radicals and help prevent oxidation and cell destruction.

Dr. Masquelier discussed the free-radical scavenging benefits of proanthocyanadins in 1986. PCOs are incorporated within the cell structure and offer defense against free-radical damage and accelerate delivery of vitamins to cells.

Another characteristic of PCOs is their ability to bind with phosphatidylcholine produced from the combination of one part grape seed and two parts lecithin. The end result is a new molecule encased by the phosphatidylcholine molecules. Not only are these molecules superior free radical scavengers, they facilitate the absorption of nutrients.

In a like manner, PCOs help to bind collagen and elasticin together. Collagen is the most abundant protein in the body and is responsible for the maintenance of tendons, ligaments, and cartilage. Collagen also helps to support the structure of the dermis and the blood vessels. By realigning the collagen fibers to a more youthful, undamaged structure, elasticity and flexibility are returned to connective tissue.

In animal trials, PCOs have been shown to lower seriously high cholesterol levels while reducing cholesterol deposits in the arteries. Therefore, it is only fair to assume that PCOs might have a similar impact in the human body.

Proanthocyanadins have demonstrated their effectiveness against cardiovascular problems, varicose veins, muscular degeneration, and diabetic retinopathy. Studies also show that PCOs might be beneficial to those who suffer from arthritis. Good clinical work is currently underway to scientifically study PCO medical value to victims of stroke and heart disease.

Poor air, polluted water, processed foods and high fat diets have all been linked to the aging process. To counteract their damaging impacts, it is estimated that you should take one 50 mg capsule of grape-seed extract for every 50 pounds of body weight. In addition to Emerald Greens, I take two to four a day because my work takes me into smog-bound Los Angeles. Grape-seed extract is vital to good cellular health.

Miracle SUPER FOODS That Heal

16. Green Tea Catechins
Tea Leaves

10 Milligrams (Mg)
in one serving (3 teaspoons) of Emerald Greens

Fact:
Green tea contains the flavonoid, quercetin, a potent antioxidant, which in medical studies decreased deaths from heart disease and risk of stroke.

When you think of tea, you probably think of England. The British Isles are synonymous with tea drinking. In 1657, tea was offered for sale at a coffeehouse in London, England, and since then, drinking a cup of tea has become part of the English way of life. There are many varieties of teas, but for the purpose of this book, our focus is on green tea, which is especially popular in Asia.

Tea started in China about 4,000 years ago. But by 1211, tea drinking had become popular in Japan thanks to a gentlemen named Eisai Myoan, founder of Zen Buddhism. Eisai wrote a book about tea and extolled its many health benefits. Eisai recounted the story of a top government official who got very sick. When Eisai instructed him to drink green tea, the officer miraculously recovered. Soon, the demand for green tea spread like wildfire throughout Japan. Eventually, tea made its way to Europe and ultimately to the rest of the world.

In Japan, the Shizuoka region produces green tea and has the lowest incidence of cancer. This fact intrigued the Japanese Department of Health, which discovered residents drank far more cups of green tea than the rest of the population. After extensive research, scientists concluded that green tea was responsible for the low incidence of cancer in both men and women in that region.

Another interesting fact is that the Japanese have the highest smoking rate of any nation. Yet, lung disease is the lowest for any developed country. Japanese men have less than one-third the number of lung cancers found in American males. It seems that green tea might also inhibit the damage inflicted by cigarette smoking.

Miracle SUPER FOODS That Heal

Only recently have scientists isolated a remarkable catechin in green tea that seems to prevent cancer in laboratory animals. This incredible substance is called epigallocatechin gallate (EGCG) and was described in 1998 by Lester Mitscher, Ph.D. Epigallocatechin gallate is a free-radical scavenger that neutralizes dietary carcinogens and dangerous reactive molecules that attack DNA and subsequently trigger cancer. ECGC also inhibits the formation of urokinase, an enzyme that aids cancer growth.

According to Dr. Fujiki of the National Cancer Center in Japan, mice given EGCG showed significant tumor reduction, which seemed linked to ECGC's ability to block carcinogens in the mice systems. Also, research from China confirmed that green tea blocks carcinogenic nitrosamines from nitrates found in processed meat. Nitrates are a known cause of stomach cancer. In another study at Rutgers University, New Jersey, mice with stomach and lung cancer were given green tea. The result was a 63% reduction in tumors.

Other active agents in green tea are called polyphenols, powerful antioxidants that protect the cells from free radical molecules such as superoxide and hydrogen peroxide. Nearly every kind of tea has at least some polyphenols, but due to the more gentle processing of green tea leaves, a greater percentage of polyphenols are retained compared to other more harshly processed teas.

In one study, for instance, green tea increased antioxidant levels in the blood six times more than black tea. In another recent study in which green tea and vitamin E were compared, green tea provided two hundred times more antioxidant protection than vitamin E. It is now known that catechin EGCG is destroyed during the production of black teas.

Green tea also has an amino acid called theanine which reputedly gives green tea its delightful taste. Cancer researchers report that thea-nine both enhances the effectiveness of several cancer medications while reducing their side effects. Therefore, green tea is used before, during, and after chemotherapy and radiation treatments for cancer patients. People who suffer from skin cancer and cancers of the esophagus, stomach and intestine, lungs, liver, prostate, bladder, and pancreas all report feeling better when they take green tea with their treatments. Other amino acids found in green tea beyond theanine are aspartic acid, glutamic acid, glutamine, tyrosine, and proline.

Green tea's benefits go beyond blocking cancer cell growth. It provides relief for individuals who suffer from heart disease, stroke, hypertension, high cholesterol, diabetes, viral and bacterial infections, and it helps to control pH levels in the colon. It even kills plaque and bacteria in the mouth, which might help prevent tooth decay.

Green tea is also full of vitamins, minerals, and amino acids. It contains vitamins such as B-2 and vitamin K and the minerals chromium, calcium, magnesium, manganese, iron, copper, zinc, phosphorus, and potassium. Most surprising of all, green tea can even be used externally. Green tea face washes contribute to healthy skin. Feet calluses and sores benefit greatly from a poultice of green tea leaves. Cold green tea bags relieve sore and tired eyes. Green tea can even be used as a hair shampoo!

However, women who are pregnant or have fibrocystic problems should avoid drinking green tea to avoid its caffeine.

Since any of us can receive thousands of free radical attacks daily from our polluted environment, it is important to keep our antioxidant levels as high as possible. If a body is out of balance and has low antioxidant protection, free-radical damage is inevitable. Green tea is one of the most powerful antioxidants we can use. The catechins in green tea neutralize free radicals before they get a chance to damage DNA.

For an in-depth study about how to use green tea to prevent cancer and slow the aging process, I recommend the marvelous book by Lester A. Mitscher, Ph.D., and Victoria Dolby entitled, *The Green Tea Book: China's Fountain of Youth*.

17. Lecithin
Soybeans (99% Oil Free)

2000 Milligrams (Mg)
in one serving (3 teaspoons) of Emerald Greens

Fact:
Lecithin is a natural emulsifier found in eggs, which is rich
in choline that moves cholesterol through the bloodstream,
aids fat metabolism, and is an essential component of cell
membranes and nerve tissue.

Lecithin, derived from the Greek word *lekithos* which means "egg yolk," is one of the building blocks of life. It exists naturally in plants and animals, especially egg yolks, corn, and soybeans. Lecithin is rich in choline needed for healthy brains. Thirty percent of brain matter in dry weight is lecithin. Human livers also synthesize choline. Our bodies use lecithin and choline as a brain tonic, to break down and metabolize fat and cholesterol, and to strengthen cell membranes.

Fats and oils are a very important part of a daily diet. But since oil and water don't mix, it takes the lecithin molecule to bind them together for processing in the body. A lecithin molecule is a bi-polar molecule. That means one end contains fatty acids attracted to oil. At the other end is phosphorus and nitrogen, which are attracted to water. Lecithin can keep fatty substances in a clean liquid state as they make their way through the watery world of blood and plasma in arteries. As long as lecithin is doing its job, dangerously thick fat deposits will not build up on blood vessel walls.

In the bloodstream, lecithin helps to prevent cholesterol and other fat build-up along the walls of arteries. At the same time, it helps dissolve fat that might already be on its way to clogging arteries. The liver is responsible for cleaning fat out of blood and can become overwhelmed and diseased if there is too much fat to process. Lecithin breaks down and metabolizes fat that can cause liver degeneration.

Lecithin in the intestinal tract assists with the absorption of fat-soluble vitamins such as A, D, E, and K. In its ability to distribute body

Miracle SUPER FOODS That Heal

fats, lecithin provides support to the nervous system and adds vitality to hair and skin.

In the brain, choline in lecithin is transformed into acetylcholine, which is necessary for nerve endings to transmit messages. Thus, lecithin and its choline transformation to acetylcholine improves memory, thinking ability, and muscle control.

Scientists have discovered that there is a blood barrier that protects the brain from toxins. Alcohol and drugs are only a few of the chemicals that are known to cross that barrier. It has now been discovered that, once lecithin is consumed, its choline is able to cross the blood-brain barrier and have a powerful effect on the production of brain chemical signals. Without lecithin, the complex control processes between the brain, nerves, and organs would not be possible.

18. Licorice Root
Glycyrrhiza glabra
Glucomannan Root Powder

20 Milligrams (Mg)
in one serving (3 teaspoons) of Emerald Greens

Fact:
Two thousand years ago, the licorice root was one of a
select group of herbs listed in the renowned Chinese
Shennong Herbal. Today among Asian healers, licorice is
highly regarded as a treatment for ulcers, arthritis,
and even cancer.

Glykyrrhiza, a slightly different spelling, is Greek for "sweet root."
You might have enjoyed licorice candy as a kid. The source of its unique
taste is licorice root, also known as sweetwood, Spanish juice root, or lick
weed. Licorice grows throughout Spain, Greece, Southern Italy, Russia,
and northern China.

Growers know that in the autumn of a licorice plant's fourth year,
the roots are at their sweetest. So that's when the root is usually harvested, cleaned, washed, trimmed, assorted in sizes, and cut up. Licorice root
is sold in bundles, bales, and bags to make elixirs, powders, syrups, tinctures, and candies.

The Russian version of licorice tends to be more popular, presum-
ably because it contains more of the active compound glycyrrhizin.
Glycyrrhizin (glycyrrhizic acid) is about fifty times sweeter than sugar cane.
Strangely, although most sugary sweets increase thirst, licorice will not.

Licorice root has been used to treat maladies for thousands of years.
It is full of vitamins and minerals including vitamin E, B-complex, phosphorus, biotin, niacin, pantothenic acid, lecithin, manganese, iodine,
chromium, and zinc. Licorice is perhaps the only herb claimed to benefit all twelve meridians in Chinese medicine. Partly due to its sweet taste,
licorice is one of the oldest and most effective remedies for constipation
in children.

When chewed or sucked, licorice root helps to increase the body's flow of saliva and mucus. It also helps to soften, soothe, nourish, and lubricate the intestinal tract, helps heal gastric ulcers, and can provide relief for bowel and urinary tract complaints.

Licorice contains glycosides that gently purge chemical debris from the lungs, throat, and body. The melting, soothing qualities of licorice in the mouth help people who suffer from bronchitis, sore throat, hoarseness, wheezing, and chest or lung problems. Licorice is also a comfort to sufferers of catarrhal nose and throat infections.

Licorice stimulates the adrenal glands and inhibits the breakdown of adrenal hormones in the liver. Professional athletes often chew on a stick of licorice because it seems to balance blood sugar levels and boost energy.

For women, licorice helps to make the female hormone estrogen because it contains phytosterols needed for the production of estrogens.

Licorice also seems to help reduce age spots, arteriosclerosis, arthritis circulatory problems, colds, drug withdrawal, emphysema, fevers, flu, and hemorrhoids.

One note of caution: licorice root might cause sodium retention and thus contribute to high blood pressure in some people. However, Emerald Greens has a low sodium to potassium ratio and is rich in magnesium and potassium which help to reduce high blood pressure.

19. Milk Thistle
Silybum marianum
Silymarin Seeds 83.5%

50 Milligrams (Mg)
in one serving (3 teaspoons) of Emerald Greens

Fact:
In European medical studies, alcoholic patients suffering from cirrhosis damage in the liver lived longer if given silymarin than those given a placebo.

Named for the milky juice its leaves emit when crushed, milk thistle is also known as Mary Thistle, Lady Thistle, or Holy Thistle. For at least the last 2,000 years, milk thistle has been the primary herb used to treat liver disorders. In the 18th Century, an herbalist named Culpepper pre- scribed the herb for obstructions of the liver and spleen.

In the 1960s, a bioflavonoid complex in milk thistle was identified. Researchers named the complex silymarin. Silymarin has three parts that are biologically active: silybin, silydianin, and silychristin. Silymarin is an antioxidant many more times powerful than vitamin E. It can block the destruction of free radicals and increase the levels of glutathione and superoxide dismutase, two of the body's own antioxidants.

Silymarin can help repair damaged liver cells and treat liver ail- ments such as jaundice and viral hepatitis. Silymarin, if given within twenty-four hours of ingestion, can even reverse potentially lethal poi- soning by amanita mushrooms.

Silymarin has been shown to change the cell structure of the outer liver membrane, which keeps toxins out and stimulates cell growth. In fact, animal studies indicate that milk thistle is able to increase the regen- eration of liver cells by a whopping four hundred to five hundred per- cent! In fact, several studies have reported that alcoholics suffering from cirrhosis have been able to repair certain liver damage by taking silymarin supplements.

Recent research in Germany indicates that silymarin prevents the depletion of antioxidants such as glutathione and superoxide dismutase in red blood cells. It also inhibits the formation of liver-damaging compounds called leukotrienes. Thus, silymarin helps to detoxify the liver, reduce nausea and boost energy and appetite.

Milk Thistle is safe and non-toxic, even for pregnant women. The recommended dosage is 200 mg two to three times daily. Its impact on improving health should be noticeable in a few weeks.

20. Probiotic Culture (Dairy Free Source)
Health-Enhancing Bacteria

135 Milligrams (Mg) or 2.5 Billion Microorganisms
in one serving (3 teaspoons) of Emerald Greens

Fact:
Each human body is host to several thousand billion
friendly bacteria, more than all the cells in your body.

Probiotic means "for life" and applies to friendly bacteria that help digestion and work together with our immune system to keep us healthy. Friendly bacteria manufacture some B vitamins, help normalize hormone levels, reduce cholesterol levels, help keep oxidizing free radicals in check, and protect us from fungi and yeasts, which can produce toxic and carcinogenic substances. As important as they are, humans often end up killing these friendly bacteria with corticosteroids, birth control pills, and antibiotics.

The most common probiotic culture is yogurt, a dairy product, which has bacteria that help, not hurt, human digestive tracts. One example of a friendly bacteria is acidophilus, which helps production of lactase enzymes in the intestines. The lactase enzymes digest lactose from dairy foods which results in lactic acid. Acidophilus and other dairy-free cultures have been shown to have a positive antimicrobial effect against infectious pathogens such as *E. coli, Candida albicans,* and salmonella.

The history behind probiotic cultures began with Nobel prize laureate Elie Metchnikoff. He was working at the Pasteur Institute in 1908 when he observed that a large number of people who resided in Bulgaria had long life spans. Metchnikoff learned that the the most common diet in that country consisted mostly of vegetables and yogurt. Since vegetables are prevalent throughout the world, they did not seem a logical answer to longevity. So, Metchnikoff studied yogurt.

Many years earlier, Louis Pasteur had discovered a way to hinder lactic fermentation that spoiled milk quickly. He heated milk just enough to kill bacteria in what became known as the pasteurization process. Then he made an unexpected discovery. Spoiled milk was full of little microbes

Miracle SUPER FOODS That Heal

called lactobacilli, which are good for you, and nutritious yogurt was born.

Later, Metchnikoff was the first researcher to prove the ability of lactobacilli to transform lactose into lactic acid. He assumed that any acid produced would be a hostile, killing environment for bacteria. In fact, many dangerous disease-producing organisms do die in milk that contains lactobacilli.

Lactobacilli are important to healthy colons, but pathogens in food and antibiotics can disrupt or destroy lactobacilli. Therefore, sometimes it is necessary to take lactobacilli supplements.

A 1976 study in Kenya, Africa showed a link between lactobacilli levels and cholesterol. The Masai tribe in Kenya has long mixed blood and milk to drink. In the controlled study, when lactobacilli were added to the Masai milk, there was a measurable reduction in the tribe's serum cholesterol levels.

Yogurt produced a similar result in a 1979 American study. Further, when mice and rats were fed acidophilus for thirty days in an Oklahoma lab, their cholesterol levels dropped twenty-three percent.

People who suffer from osteoporosis might also benefit from lactobacilli. The reason is that the bacteria enhance calcium absorption, which is vital for building bone tissue and preventing bone loss. Lactobacilli also help balance blood sugar levels which is valuable to diabetics.

Lactobacilli enhance mineral absorption. The bacteria aid protein digestion and the assimilation of vitamins and other nutrients. Adding lactobacilli supplements to a diet means that B vitamins are more easily manufactured, nitrogen retention is enhanced, carbohydrates are fermented, and fatty acids are more efficiently removed from fat reserves.

Lactobacilli help reduce vitamin and mineral deficiencies, skin problems, liver toxins, digestive disorders, diarrhea, cancer, and even halitosis, or bad breath.

Lactobacilli come in different preparations such as capsules, tablets, powders, or freeze-dried. The most effective storage seems to be freeze-dried since that process does the least damage to the bacteria. Whatever form you use, it should always be refrigerated after opening. Store the product in dark bottles to protect the fragile bacteria from sunlight.

The best time to ingest these friendly bacteria is at least one to two hours before a meal and then with water only. Emerald Greens contains 2.5 billion lactobacilli per serving.

21. Royal Jelly
The Nutritious Nectar of Queen Bees
3.3X Honeycomb Concentrate

60 Milligrams (Mg)
in one serving (3 teaspoons) of Emerald Greens

Fact:
The queen bee in a hive is fed royal jelly, a white, milky secretion produced by worker bees that is a complete protein, containing all essential amino acids and B vitamins. The queen grows to be 50% larger, lives up to 40 times longer, and is highly fertile compared to the worker bees who don't eat royal jelly.

Queen bees are born from the exact same eggs as worker bees. The subsequent difference is that only queen bees are fed exclusively with royal jelly secreted by the pharyngeal glands of nurse bees. This diet enables the queen to grow approximately forty to sixty percent larger than worker bees. Eventually she will produce 2.5 times her own body weight in eggs every single day. Perhaps most amazing of all, the queen bee lives four to five times longer than her genetically identical sisters who are not fed royal jelly.

Royal jelly is a super food that is twelve percent protein and contains:
- Eight B vitamins (B-1, B-2, B-5, B-6, B-12, Biotin, folic acid, and pantothenic acid) are known for their ability to reduce stress levels.
- Twenty-two amino acids, including the eight most essential required for good health such as aspartic acid, which aids tissue growth.
- Gamma globulin, which boosts the immune system to fight infections.
- Minerals such as calcium, copper, iron, phosphorus, potassium, silicon, and sulfur.

Half the total fatty acid content of royal jelly consists of a mysterious compound called 10-hydroxy-2-decanoic acid, or 10-HDA. Researchers tell us that it may be responsible for the queen bee's exceptional size and fertility. According to Japanese scientists, 10-HDA might possess antibacterial and antibiotic properties. Further studies are currently underway to determine if it is valuable in cancer prevention.

There are no solvents used in the manufacturing of royal jelly so that people with a chemical sensitivity will not have problems consuming royal jelly.

In its natural state, royal jelly contains sixty-six percent moisture by weight. Proper storage is then vitally important because it can go rancid easily. Fresh royal jelly should always be kept frozen unless it is blended into proper amounts of honey. The royal jelly in Emerald Greens is freeze-dried into a powder, which helps ensure its potency.

22. Siberian "Ginseng" Root
Eleutherococcus senticosus

80 Milligrams (Mg)
in one serving (3 teaspoons) of Emerald Greens

Fact:
The biologically active ingredients in Siberian "ginseng" are
eleutherosides shown in some studies to increase energy
and alertness, relieve stress, strengthen immune function,
and inhibit cancer tumor growth in animals.

Siberian "ginseng" is technically not ginseng. Its botanical grouping is *Eleutherococcus senticosus,* not the *Panax* species of true ginsengs. However, Siberian ginseng has many of the same chemical effects as true ginseng and is usually cheaper to buy. The ginseng root that grows in China has been used as a cure-all for most medical problems. In fact, the generic name of the plant, *Panax,* is derived from Greek meaning "panacea," or cure-all. North American Indians considered the ginseng root sacred.

The name ginseng comes from the Chinese words that mean "man" and "slippery root." The root resembles the human body and has a smooth skin. The first mention of ginseng can be found in the earliest Chinese herb book, the *Pen Tsao Ching.* According to Chinese legend, ginseng should be taken for a wise, long life. Poetically, it is used for calming the spirit, curtailing emotions and agitations, removing noxious influences, brightening eyes, lifting the mind, and increasing wisdom.

Ginseng grows wild in two parts of the world, Asia and North America. Ideal growing conditions for ginseng are humid summers and winter temperatures that drop below freezing. The best harvest time is when the plant is five or six years old and its root's active ingredients are at their peak.

There are several different species in the ginseng family including Oriental ginseng (*Panax ginseng*), wild American ginseng (*Panax quinquefolium*), dwarf ginseng (*Panax trifotius*), sanchi ginseng (*Panax nitoginseng*), Himalayan ginseng (*Panax pseudoginseng*), Japanese ginseng (*Panax*

Miracle SUPER FOODS That Heal

Japanicus), Brazilian ginseng known as Suma, which relieves pain and regulates hormones, women's ginseng (*Dong quai*) used to regulate menstrual problems, and the popular Siberian "ginseng" (*Eleutherococcus senticosus*). There is much debate about which ginseng is best for which malady. Siberian ginseng, not truly a ginseng, lasts longer than true ginsengs, is somewhat more soothing, and is less expensive.

All ginsengs contain a rich assortment of vitamins and minerals such as A, B-1, B-2, B-12, pantothenic acid, biotin, vitamin E, zinc, manganese, calcium, iron, and copper. California ginseng is used to treat lung problems, prevent thirst, and increase energy. Oregon ginseng historically has been used to treat pain, rheumatism, and obesity. Indian ginseng, also known as Ashwaganda, is used to treat insomnia, impotence, and old age.

Russian and Japanese scientists have carried out the most extensive research on ginseng. The researchers agree that ginsengs contain remarkable compounds, which the Japanese call ginsenosides and the Russians call panaxosides. Russian research indicates that, when the body is under stress, Siberian ginseng promotes rapid corticosteroid release to return systems to their more normal, less stressed states.

Japanese scientists reported in the U. S. *Journal of Cancer Research* that Oriental ginseng (*Panax ginseng*) not only stopped the growth of malignant liver cells in test tubes, but even returned diseased cells to normal, both in terms of function and shape. According to the scientists, once-cancerous cells now resembled "original normal liver cells."

Upon further study, the Japanese discovered that a single chemical found in ginseng known as ginsenosdie rh2 could revert melanoma skin cancer cells back to normal. Additional research indicated an immune-boosting effect on white blood cells in cancer patients.

Russian, German, and American researchers have discovered that ginseng raises interferon production, which helps to protect cells against viral infections. Leukocytes in the blood are dramatically reduced once ginsenosides enter the bloodstream. A high leukocyte level normally indicates an infection is present.

Perhaps the most celebrated quality of ginseng is its ability to boost energy. Ginseng improves endurance, respiration, oxygen consumption, and muscle strength, and helps the heart muscle stay healthy. Thus, ginseng is particularly helpful for chronic fatigue sufferers.

In one case study, ginseng supplements were used for about one month and oxygen intake increased by twenty-nine percent. In another controlled study performed by the Italian researcher, Dr. H. Quiroga, those who took a ginseng tincture increased blood flow to their brains by thirty-four percent.

What's more, ginseng is probably the most powerful herb in the production of Adenosine Triphosphate (ATP), which is a small molecule that stores energy and drives chemical reactions in the body.

Professional athletes will be interested to learn that ginseng prevents overworked muscles from cramping and soreness and might help muscles recover more rapidly by reducing the amount of lactic acid in the blood. The powerful antioxidants in ginseng help to counteract free radicals and other scavengers which cause oxidation during rigorous exercise.

Due to its beneficial effect on the circulatory system, ginseng has often been used to treat heart disease. Ginseng increases blood flow, reduces blood pressure and slows heart rate, lowers cholesterol, and reduces risk of blood clots. Researchers believe that ginseng, combined with medication, might be able to strengthen blood vessels to counteract degeneration and arteriosclerosis, especially in the elderly.

Ginseng is particularly good for brain cell stimulation. In Europe, it is commonly used to treat those who suffer from depression. It makes the eyes more responsive to light and improves night vision. Ginseng is also known to improve hearing and mental concentration.

The Chinese also believe ginseng improves virility, restores sexual energy, and invigorates pregnant women. Hot flashes due to hormonal imbalances at menopause are usually reduced or entirely disappear for most women when given ginseng.

Reports from China indicate that blood-sugar levels in diabetics treated with ginseng dropped forty to fifty percent. Chinese doctors also use ginseng to treat arthritis, alcoholism, and liver disease. It's also thought that cancer patients undergoing radiation treatments can benefit greatly from consuming ginseng.

Externally, ginseng is used by many women as a rejuvenating, moisturizing face cream. It seems to replenish and restore damaged skin and might reduce the appearance of wrinkles. Ginseng flowers and leaves are used medicinally as teas and sometimes as a tonic for baths.

Ginseng comes in many forms and you need to find what works best for you. Emerald Greens has ginseng in powder form which is easy for the

Miracle SUPER FOODS That Heal

body to assimilate. There are many ginsengs other than those mentioned in this book, so if you purchase ginseng separately, look for a product that is standardized. For example, the brand China White sells for around $60/pound. Red Ginseng is very popular and sells for $85 to $150/pound.

Scientific studies confirm that ginseng is non-toxic and can be used safely and effectively for the long term as long as it is not taken together with medications or coffee. The reason is that such combinations might be too stimulating for the central nervous system. It is also wise to consult your physician or health care professional before taking ginseng if you have high blood pressure or diabetes. Otherwise, ginseng is a safe and effective super food.

23. Spirulina Powder
Blue Green Algae

1000 Milligrams (Mg)
in one serving (3 teaspoons) of Emerald Greens

Fact:
Green vegetables from the land or sea are excellent sources
of complex carbohydrates, dietary fiber, beta-carotene, and
chlorophyll and contain powerful antioxidants which
destroy free radicals and help fight cancer.

Spirulina is a single-celled blue-green algae which has thrived in warm climates on this earth for some 3.5 billion years. Ideal growing temperatures range from 85 degrees to 100 degrees Fahrenheit. There are many different varieties that grow in oceans and lakes.

Some scientists have described spirulina as Nature's most complete food and a boon for vegetarians. Spirulina is comprised of sixty-five percent easily digestible protein, ten to fifteen percent carbohydrates (primarily rhamnose and glycogen, and some sugar.

Both rhamnose and glycogen are polysaccharides, which are easily absorbed by the body without triggering a lot of insulin. Therefore, spirulina can provide quick energy boosts without burdening the pancreas, which helps people with blood sugar problems such as hypoglycemia.

Spirulina also supplies liberal amounts of vitamins, minerals, nucleic acids, and ten of the twelve non-essential amino acids, which complement the essential amino acids that are the building blocks of proteins. For instance, spirulina is a rich source of vitamin B-12, essential fatty acids, and iron. It contains ten times the beta-carotene concentration found in carrots. Furthermore, spirulina contains a large number of enzymes that are necessary for the breakdown of fats, proteins, and carbohydrates.

In Japan, where spirulina has long been part of the daily diet, medical practitioners have been documenting the positive effects spirulina has had on individuals with chronic fatigue and other debilitating diseases. Spirulina, like several of the other super foods, contains the antioxidant superoxide dismutase, an enzyme that protects the body from free radical scavengers. It is also high in chlorophyll, which helps detoxify the entire gastrointestinal tract. Spirulina has been used successfully in the treatment of diabetes, anemia, liver disease, ulcers, allergies, radiation poisoning, chemical poisoning, and senility.

Spirulina has also helped obese patients cut down food intake. Dr. Richard Passwater says that the amino acid structure of spirulina might directly influence levels of neurotransmitters in the brain, particularly those that control appetite, ambition, and mood. He goes on to say that it is the high concentration of the amino acid phenylalanine that seems to alter brain chemistry so that appetite cravings are not so dominant.

Where countries don't have enough food, spirulina could also help the hungry. Forty to sixty million people each year starve to death; 1.3 billion go to bed each night with empty stomachs. Shockingly, empty stomachs and poor nutrition kill forty to sixty thousand children in the prosperous United States each year. Yet, there is enough spirulina growing along the pristine coast of Kona, Hawaii, for example, to feed all the hungry children worldwide.

Miracle SUPER FOODS That Heal

24. Suma Powder
Brazilian "Ginseng" Dried Root
(*Pfaffia paniculata*)

60 Milligrams (Mg)
in one serving (3 teaspoons) of Emerald Greens

Fact:
Suma root contains allantoin, which stimulates protein synthesis and boosts immune function. The root also has cancer-fighting substances called pfaffosides, which can inhibit growth of melanoma cells in lab culture dishes.

Suma bark and root have been used for three centuries in South America as a tonic to increase a sense of well being. Miners who work three hundred feet down in South American mine shafts use suma for endurance. The Portuguese call it "Para Todo," which means "for everything."

Suma is an adaptogen, a name used to describe any substance that enables the body to better cope with stress. Suma boosts immune responses to microbes and could help AIDS and other patients whose immune systems are weak. Japanese researchers report that saponins called pfaffosides in suma chemistry can inhibit cultured melanoma tumor cells in laboratory Petri dishes.

Another compound in suma is called allantoin, which is known to promote new cell growth and healing of wounds.

Suma also contains phytosterols such as beta-ecdysone. Beta-ecdysone is a plant hormone that enhances protein synthesis and creation of living tissues.

Two other plant hormones found in suma are sitosterol and stipmasterol. These phytochemicals nourish the circulatory and glandular systems. Both have been found to increase circulation and reduce cholesterol levels in the blood. Sitosterol also interferes with destructive free-radical movement in the body and enhances production of estrogen.

If you suffer from anemia, stress, high blood pressure, or liver problems, suma could be a positive addition to your diet. Suma helps to restore sexual functions and protect the body against viral infections. Suma has also been shown to be beneficial in the treatment of diabetes, digestion, and skin problems. Professional athletes around the world use suma before competitions because it purportedly increases stamina.

Suma contains a full range of amino acids and a rare mineral salt called germanium which helps oxygen flow to cells. Other minerals in suma include iron, magnesium, phosphorous, potassium, copper, and calcium. Its vitamin content includes A, B-1, B-2, C, D, E, and K.

Suma extract is non-toxic, has no known side effects, and comes in powder, drops, or capsules.

25. Wheat Grass Juice Powder (Organic)
Wheat Leaves

430 Milligrams (Mg)
in one serving (3 teaspoons) of Emerald Greens

Fact:
Green foods such as young wheat grass are high in
vitamins, minerals, enzymes, fiber, and chlorophyll,
the "blood" of plants.

Nearly half of all the cultivated land on our planet is used to grow cereal grains. One third of that total is planted in wheat. Wheat grass was a staple of the Greeks and Romans at least 3,000 years ago.

Wheat grass is wheat that has been harvested just before the green plant germinates into golden stalks of grain, known as the jointing stage. The wheat plants must accumulate high levels of energy to accomplish that transformation, so the jointing stage is when wheat nutrients are at their peak.

In the late 1960s, wheat grass juice became part of the health food movement. These days, it is in health food stores everywhere. Some stores sell wheat grass juice by the glass.

Wheat grass contains an abundance of chlorophyll, the pigment that gives plants their green color and is rich in magnesium. As I pointed out earlier in the book, the chlorophyll molecule contains the same ring structure. At the center of the hemoglobin rings is a single atom of iron. At the center of the chlorophyll's is a single atom of magnesium. In other words, both are "bloods" — green for plants and red for animals.

Wheat grass has been thoroughly researched by Dr. Ann Wigmore in her book, *Why Suffer?* Dr. Wigmore wrote that wheat grass grown in good soil up to about six inches in height absorbs minerals, vitamins, and trace elements which have a total acid content that comes very close to pH 7.4, the slightly alkaline chemistry of healthy human blood.

Famed nutritionist Dr. Bernard Jenson applauds the benefits of fresh wheat grass juice and its chlorophyll because of the high enzymatic activity. He states, "It takes hours of energy to digest solid food, but only

Miracle SUPER FOODS That Heal

minutes and very little energy for the body to assimilate chlorophyll."

Chlorophyll is produced when sunshine falls on plants. It is known to have revitalizing, regenerative, and detoxifying effects on humans. By increasing oxygenation in the body, foods high in chlorophyll can help counteract living in a polluted world of smog and carbon monoxide.

Well known for its blood-cleansing abilities, the chlorophyll in wheat grass helps to wash drug deposits from the body. Recent research also indicates that wheat grass juice might even offset the damaging effects of radiation and x-rays. In scientific studies, chlorophyll has demonstrated an ability to nourish the intestines and to soothe and heal the mucous lining. For years, dentists have used chlorophyll to successfully treat oral diseases from tooth decay to pyorrhea, while physicians have used it to treat kidney stones and infections of the upper respiratory tract and sinuses.

The health benefits of wheat grass extend far beyond its rich chlorophyll content. Wheat grass contains high amounts of proteins and a larger amount of essential amino acids than other plants. Vegetarians should take note that wheat grass has more protein than eggs.

Wheat grass juice powder is rich in vitamins C and K and many of the B vitamins. It contains a total of 90 minerals which include calcium, iron, magnesium, phosphorus, potassium, sodium, sulphur, cobalt, and zinc.

Wheat grass is also a good source of beta-carotene, which is converted by the body into vitamin A as needed. A 1982 report from the National Academy of Sciences, entitled "Diet, Nutrition and Cancer Status," revealed that "epidemiological research is sufficient to suggest that foods rich in carotene are associated with a reduced risk of cancer." Those foods include carrots and wheat grass.

Wheat grass consumption is good for the heart, lungs, intestines, uterus, and vascular system. It has been used in the treatment of such diverse ailments as a sore throat, arthritis, leukemia, and emphysema.

Besides being a cancer-preventive agent, wheat grass is an effective immune stimulator, which helps the body fight infections. Wheat grass juice also kills germs when applied to cuts and bruises. Juiced wheat grass can also be used as a skin cleanser, to treat acne, eczema, and psoriasis, and even as a hair tonic to treat dandruff and keep hair from graying.

For constipation sufferers, wheat grass aids digestion, and adds high fiber and magnesium to the system.

How much wheat grass should one consume? It is best to start slowly, usually no more than one ounce, and build up to six ounces a day. Sip the juice, mix thoroughly with your saliva, and drink slowly. Some people experience nausea when they first take wheat grass. Add a little water and very gently ease your way into it. Wheat grass is best taken at least one hour before meals and two hours after. Emerald Greens contains 430 mg. of wheat grass chlorophyll per serving.

Miracle SUPER FOODS That Heal

26. Wheat Sprout Powder
Wheat Sprouts

300 Milligrams (Mg)
in one serving (3 teaspoons) of Emerald Greens

Fact:
One cup of raw wheat sprouts contains eight grams of
protein and three milligrams each of vitamin C and niacin,
plus folacin, riboflavin, and trace minerals.

Some 30,000 varieties of wheat are grown throughout the world. Newly sprouted seedlings must absorb a lot of water to grow. In so doing, the rapidly developing sprouts must also create large concentrations of antioxidant enzymes to protect themselves from free radicals in the water.

Botanists have capitalized on this trait by developing several strains of enzyme-rich super sprouts germinated from specially bred wheat. Dried at low temperatures using special enzyme-preserving techniques, each strain of super sprouts emphasizes a specific antioxidant enzyme complex. Since antioxidant enzymes work synergistically with other cellular materials, antioxidant enzymes remove free radicals up to ten times faster than antioxidant vitamins and minerals alone.

Wheat sprouts can enhance the body's own production of antioxidant enzymes, including glutathione peroxidase, methione reductase, catalase, and that important superoxide dismutase mentioned frequently in the contents of other super foods.

Scientists tell us that the life span of man and many animals is proportional to the level of superoxide dismutase in the brain, heart, and liver. The reason is that superoxide dismutase is very effective in preventing and repairing DNA damage. Unfortunately, by the time we reach eighty, our level of superoxide dismutase will have dropped from roughly 1700 units per gram of body weight to approximately 50 units. This large drop in enzyme levels allows unstable free-radical molecules to steal electrons from other molecules, wreaking havoc on healthy cells.

Wheat sprouts are a rich source of antioxidant enzymes that help maintain cellular integrity and thwart free-radical chain reactions before they get out of control.

Emerald Greens has an abundance of wheat sprout enzymes. If longevity and healthy living are what you seek, add wheat sprouts to your daily diet.

"For the earth bringeth forth fruit of herself; first the blade, then the ear, after that the full corn in the ear."

Mark 4:28

"Let food be your medicine."

Hippocrates

Testimonials

One of my greatest joys is to receive cards and letters every day from customers who tell me what a difference Emerald Greens has made in their lives. I would like to share with you some of their first-hand experiences.

"Dear Tony,

Your product Emerald Greens must be magic! After two days on the product, I could get by without reading glasses in the pharmacy. I got used to reading expiration dates on containers, prescriptions and so on without glasses. I ran out of Emerald Greens (and then) two days later, I can't see without the reading glasses. Needless to say, I reordered your product and again two days on and my sight is back. I will never run out of Emerald Greens again. Besides improving my vision, it also curbs my appetite. What a bonus!

Emerald Greens is my answer to better nutrition. My work schedule hardly allows time to plan a balanced diet. With Emerald Greens, I get my vitamins, minerals, enzymes, fiber, anti-oxidants and amino acids. This product represents a major step towards better nutrition in a very palatable fruit juice. This is the super food of the 90s! I'm so glad I discovered it."

Karen Knoke, R. Ph.
Las Vegas, Nevada

"Dear Tony,

My name is John Howie. I am a C6-7 quadriplegic. I have been in a wheelchair for 12 years. I am writing because several months ago I purchased some Emerald Greens. Up until that point, I had been experiencing urinary tract infections every six to eight weeks (a common occurrence among quads). I am very pleased to report that since I got Emerald Greens, I have not had a single infection, with the exception of one week when I forgot to take them with me and sure enough, I got an infection. Thank you very much for your quality product."

John Howie
Monroe, North Carolina

"Dear Tony,

Just a few words of praise about Emerald Greens:
One of our employees tested positive for HIV and usually missed four to five days a week. He is on his second bottle (of Emerald Greens) and has not missed a day since he began taking it.

My brother has prostate cancer that has spread to his back. He has been taking Emerald Greens for over one year in addition to other treatments and is able to work. He attributes his energy to Emerald Greens."

Patricia Shepard
San Buenaventura, California

Emerald Greens SUPER FOODS Ingredients

Super Food	Amount Per One Serving (3 Tsp)
1. Acerola Berry Juice Powder (Vit. C)	100 Mgs from berries.
2. Apple Pectin	670 Mgs from fruit.
3. Apple Fiber	670 Mgs from fruit.
4. Alfalfa Juice Powder (Organic)	430 Mgs from leaves.
5. Astragalus Root	80 Mgs from root.
6. Barley Grass Leaf Juice Powder	430 Mgs from leaves.
7. Barley Malt (Organic)	300 Mgs from seeds.
8. Bee Pollen	200 Mgs from flowers.
9. Beet Juice Powder	250 Mgs from root.
10. Bilberry (European) Extract	10 Mgs from berries extract.
11. Brown Rice Bran	400 Mgs from seeds.
12. Chlorella (Cracked Cell)	250 Mgs from leaves cell.
13 D-Alpha Tocopherol Acetate (Vit. E)	100 IU from synthetic process.
14. Dulse from Nova Scotia	250 Mgs from sea weed herb.
15. *Echinacea augustifolia*	80 Mgs from herb.
16. *Ginkgo biloba* Extract 24%	30 Mgs from leaves extract.
17. Glucomannan Root Powder	20 Mgs from root powder.
18. Grape-Seed Extract	10 Mgs from seeds extract.
19. Green Tea Catechins	10 Mgs from leaves.
20. Lecithin Soy (99% oil free)	2000 Mgs from soy beans.
21. Oat Beta Glucan Extract	50 Mgs seed extract.
22. Probiotic Culture (Dairy-Free) 2.5	135 Mgs of microorganisms.
23. Royal Jelly 3.3X Concentrate	60 Mgs from honeycomb.
24. Siberian Ginseng	80 Mgs from root.
25. Silymarin 83.5% (Milk Thistle)	50 Mgs from seed.
26. Spirulina Powder	1000 Mgs from blue green algae.
27. Suma Powder	60 Mgs from root.
28. Wheat Grass Juice Powder/Organic	430 Mgs from leaves.
29. Wheat Sprout Powder	300 Mgs from sprouts.

Miracle SUPER FOODS That Heal

Glossary

Acerola. A Caribbean cherry or berry rich in vitamin C.

Acid. Sour tasting liquid solution that can dissolve certain metals to form salts, or react with bases or alkalis to form salts.

Adaptogen. A substance that builds resistance to stress by strengthening the immune system, nervous system, and/or glandular system. Examples are *Echinacea*, ginseng, and *Ginkgo biloba*.

Adrenal Glands. There is one above each kidney. They secrete hormones and epinephrine, which stimulate autonomic nerve action.

Albumin. Any of several simple, water-soluble proteins that are strong antioxidants, coagulated by heat, and are found in egg white, blood serum, milk, various animal tissues, and many plant juices and tissues.

Algae. Various primitive, chiefly aquatic, one-celled or multicellular plants that lack true stems, roots, and leaves, but usually contain chlorophyll. Included among algae are kelps and other seaweeds and the diatoms.

Alkali. A hydroxide or carbonate of an alkali metal such as lithium, sodium, potassium, rubidium cesium, and francium, the aqueous solution of which is bitter, slippery, caustic, and basic in reactions.

Allylic Sulfides. Antioxidant phytochemical that stimulates production of protective enzymes; found in garlic and onions.

Amino Acids. Any organic compound containing both an amino group and a carboxylic acid group, essential for making protein molecules.

Anthrocyanin Pigments. The red, purple, and blue pigments present in fruits and vegetables such as red cabbage, beets, raspberries, red and blue plums. Colors change in presence of acids or alkalis.

Antibiotic. Any of various substances, such as penicillin and streptomycin, produced by certain fungi, bacteria, and other organisms that are capable of killing or inhibiting the growth of bacteria or other microorganisms. Widely used in disease treatment.

Antihistamine. Any of various drugs used to reduce physiological effects associated with histamine production in allergies and colds.

Antioxidants. A chemical compound or substance that inhibits oxidation. Oxidation occurs when substances interact with very reactive free radicals (single electrons separated from pairs or groups of electrons) that usually cause damage, such as cell destruction, iron rust, and dry, cracked rubber. Oxygen is an oxidant.

Arteriosclerosis. A blood circulation disorder caused by thickened and stiff artery walls, which impedes flow to and from the heart.

Aspartic Acid. A nonessential amino acid found especially in young sugar cane and sugar beet molasses that helps keep DNA and immune systems healthy.

Astragalus Root. A Chinese herb, also known as huang chi and Milk Vetch, which resembles the ball of the human ankle joint. Used medicinally to treat many disorders.

Autoimmune Disease. Any condition in which the body's immune system attacks the body's own tissues. Examples are diabetes (pancreas attacked), multiple sclerosis (nerve sheaths attacked), and rheumatoid arthritis (bone joints and cartilage attacked).

Beta-carotene. A carotenoid chemical found in plants such as carrots, yellow and orange fruits, broccoli, and spinach. The body converts beta-carotene to vitamin A, which is essential for normal eyesight, healthy tissue, a strong immune system, and bone development. Beta-carotene might reduce both the risk of cancer and cardiovascular disease. Alpha carotene, a related chemical, has been shown to suppress the growth of cancerous tumors in animals.

Betaine. A sweet, crystalline alkaloid from sugar beets and other plants used in the treatment of muscular degeneration.

Bioflavonoid. Any of a group of biologically active substances found widely in plants, which function to maintain small blood-vessel walls. Also antioxidant phytochemical which inhibits cancer-promoting hormones. Found in most fresh fruits and vegetables. "Bio" is Greek for life and "flavo" is Latin for yellow color.

Bi-polar Emulsifier Molecule. One end contains fatty acids, which can attract oil. The other end is phosphorus and nitrogen, which attract water. So these molecules can move fats through the body.

Bran. The seed husk or outer coating of cereals such as wheat, rye, rice, and oats, which contain fiber and minerals.

Capillaries. Smallest blood vessels, only one cell in diameter, which exchange nutrients and wastes between the bloodstream and the body's cells.

Carbohydrate. Any of a group of chemical compounds, including sugars, starches, and cellulose, which contain carbon, hydrogen, and oxygen only. A major source of food energy.

Complex Carbohydrate. Chemical structure that releases sugar into the blood slowly and provides fiber, such as starchy potatoes and skins.

Carcinogen. A substance that causes cells to change and can produce cancers.

Catechins (tannins). Antioxidant phytochemical found in berries and green tea.

Chlorella. Any of various blue-green algae widely used in studies of photosynthesis.

Chlorophyll. Green pigments found in photosynthetic plants. This "blood" of plants has a molecular shape similiar to human hemoglobin. There is a magnesium atom at the center of the chlorophyll molecule, but an iron atom is central to the hemoglobin molecule.

Cholesterol. A substance that is soluble in fats and is produced by all vertebrates. Necessary to create cell membranes and to transport and absorb fatty acids.

Choline. A natural amine often classed in the vitamin B complex; a precursor of acetylcholine, which makes nerve transmissions possible in the brain.

Collagen. One of two types of connective tissue (the other is elastin), which holds together tendons, cartilage, and connective tissue.

Chronic Fatigue Syndrome. An illness of chronic exhaustion that includes neurological problems such as vertigo and tunnel vision and a variety of flulike symptoms. Classified by some medical experts as an autoimmune disease.

Dietary Fiber. Indigestible food components of edible plants that the human digestive system cannot process and that add bulk and fluid to intestines, aiding contractions and elimination.

DNA. Deoxyribonucleic acid, the cell's genetic blueprint. Contains genome sequencing, which determines what any given life form and its hereditary characteristics will be.

Dulse. A coarse, reddish-brown seaweed sometimes eaten as a vegetable, from the Old Irish word *duilesc* which means "seaweed."

Echinacea. A purple-cone flowering plant used by Native Americans to treat snake bites and other skin wounds. Considered an immune booster that helps reduce cold symptoms, but does not prevent colds.

Elasticin. One of two types of connective tissue (the other is collagen), which holds together tendons, cartilage, and connective tissue.

Emulsifier. Any substance that will allow mixture of oil and water such as suspension of oily milk fats in watery milk.

Endocrine System. Ductless glands, including the thyroid, thymus, pituitary, adrenal, pancreas, ovaries, and testes, whose secretions release directly into the bloodstream.

Enzymes. Any of numerous proteins or conjugated proteins produced by living organisms, which speed chemical reactions in the body.

Epigallocatechin Gallate (EGCG). Free-radical scavenger that neutralizes dietary carcinogens and dangerous, reactive oxidizers that attack DNA and subsequently can trigger cancer. ECGC also inhibits the formation of urokinase, an enzyme that aids cancer growth. Found in green tea.

Escherichia coli (E. coli). A bacteria that traditionally has lived in benign harmony with human intestines and synthesizes B vitamins. But there is at least one killer strain of *E. coli* that has caused an increase in food poisonings from unpasteurized milk and undercooked meats, especially hamburger and hotdogs.

Essential Fatty Acids (EFAs). Any fatty acid that cannot be synthesized by the body and must be obtained from dietary sources.

Fats. Lipids easily stored in the body for fuel and cell building.

Flavonoids. Phytochemicals that make up a large group of 5,000 colorless or white to yellow pigments concentrated in the skin, rind, and outer layers of many fruits and vegetables, which have strong antioxidant properties and help plants fight disease microbes, free radicals, and other stress factors.

Folic Acid. A yellow-orange member of the vitamin-B complex that occurs in green plants, fresh fruit, liver, and yeast and is used medicinally to treat life-threatening anemias.

Free Radicals (oxidants). An atom, or group of atoms, that is highly reactive because it has at least one unpaired electron. The result is oxidation and cell destruction. Free-radical damage accelerates aging and probably contributes to many major chronic diseases. Free radicals are formed in the presence of atmospheric radiation, such as ultraviolet in sunshine, environmental pollutants, and heating fats and oils. Antioxidants bind with and neutralize free radicals.

Gamma Globulin. Any of several globulin fractions of blood serum that help the immune system fight microbes. Used to treat measles, polio, infectious hepatitis, and other infectious diseases.

Glucose. A sugar, dextrose.

Glycoside. Any of a group of organic compounds that occur abundantly in plants and produce sugars and related substances.

Glutathione Peroxidase. Antioxidant enzyme produced by human body.

Gluten. A mixture of plant proteins occurring in cereal grains, chiefly corn and wheat, and used as an adhesive and as a flour substitute.

Gram (g). One-thousandth of a kilogram (kg), or 1000 milligrams (mg).

Herb. Any plant or plant substance used primarily in medicine or food seasoning.

Homeopathy. A system of medical treatments based on the use of very small quantities of substances that in large doses would produce effects similar to the disease being treated.

Hypertension. Abnormally high arterial blood pressure.

Interferon. A cellular protein produced in response to, and acting to prevent replication of, an infectious virus within an infected cell.

Isoflavones. Antioxidant phytochemical that inhibits estrogen uptake; destroys cancer enzymes. Found in legumes such as beans, peanuts, and peas.

IU. International Unit for Vitamin A in which 3.3 International Units (IU) equal 1 Retinol Equivalent (RE) if Vitamin A source is animal; or 10 IU = 1 RE if source is plant beta-carotene.

Lactase. An enzyme in certain yeasts and in the intestinal juices of mammals that catalyzes the conversion of lactose into glucose and galactose.

Lacteal. Any of numerous tiny lymph-carrying vessels that convey chyle (lymph and emulsified fat) from the intestine to the thoracic duct.

Lactic Acid. A hygroscopic syrupy liquid present in sour milk, molasses, various fruits, and wines and used in foods and beverages to add acid, flavor, and to preserve.

Lactobacilli. Any of various types of helpful bacteria that ferment lactic acid from carbohydrates.

Lecithin. A substance found in all plant and animal tissues that is a natural emulsifier. Produced commercially from egg yolks, soybeans and corn and used in the processing of foods, pharmaceuticals, cosmetics, paints, inks, rubber, and plastics.

Leukocytes. Any of the white or colorless nucleated cells in blood that help the immune system fight off disease microbes.

Lignans. Antioxidant phytochemicals that inhibit estrogen and block prostaglandins. Found in fatty fish, flaxseed, walnuts.

Lipoprotein. A type of protein molecule that can transport lipids in the lymph and blood.

Lymph Nodes. Nodes in lymphatic vessels that supply microbe-fighting lymphocytes to the circulatory system, which remove bacteria and foreign particles from the lymph.

Macular Degeneration. The macula is part of the retina where light is focused after it passes through the lens and eyeball. Twenty percent of people over 65 will lose all or part of their vision to macular degeneration. Antioxidants that maintain retina capillary health such as *Ginko biloba* can help prevent macular degeneration.

Microgram (mcg). One millionth of a gram (g).

Milligram (mg). One-thousandth of a gram (g) or 1000 micrograms (mcg).

Minerals:

Boron - Studies indicate this mineral might help regulate the body's use of calcium, phosphorus, and magnesium. Found in fruits and vegetables, especially apples, pears, broccoli, and carrots.

Calcium - Vital to build strong bones and teeth, for muscle and nerve function, blood clotting, and metabolism. Found in milk and milk products, tofu, canned sardines and salmon, and dark green vegetables.

Chlorine (chloride) - Maintains proper body chemistry. Used to make digestive juices. Found in table salt, seafood, milk, eggs, meat.

Chromium - Works with insulin to metabolize glucose. Found in brewer's yeast, whole-grain products, liver, cheese, beer.

Copper - Component of several enzymes. Promotes iron absorption; essential to red blood cells, connective tissue, nerve fibers, and skin pigment. Found in liver, shellfish, peas, beans, nuts, and prunes.

Fluorine (fluoride) - Helps maintain strong bones and teeth. Found in tea and fluoridated water.

Germanium - A rare mineral salt that helps oxygen flow to cells and can enhance immune function, particularly in people with autoimmune diseases. Found in garlic, shiitake mushrooms, ginseng, suma, and aloe vera.

Iodine - Necessary to make thyroid hormones in thyroid gland. Found in iodized salt and seafoods.

Iron - Needed for transport and storage of oxygen in blood. Found in liver, meat, seafood, peas, beans, and fortified cereals.

Magnesium - Stimulates bone growth; necessary for muscle function and metabolism. Found in leafy green vegetables, peas, beans, whole-grain cereals and breads, meats, poultry, fish, eggs, and apricots.

Manganese - Component of many enzymes needed for metabolism; necessary to make bones and tendons. Found in coffee, tea, nuts, peas, beans and bran, vegetables and fruits.

Molybdenum - Component of enzymes needed for metabolism; instrumental in iron storage. Found in liver and other organ meats; dark green leafy vegetables, beans, and whole-grain products.

Phosphorus - Helps maintain strong bones and teeth; component of some enzymes; essential for proper metabolism. Found in meat, poultry, fish, egg yolks, peas, beans, dairy products, and soft drinks.

Potassium - Along with sodium, helps to maintain fluid balance; promotes proper metabolism and muscle function. Found in oranges, avocados, bananas, citrus and dried fruits, peas, beans, potato skins and other vegetables, yogurt, milk, whole-grain products, and meat.

Selenium - Antioxidant that works with vitamin E to protect cell membranes from oxidative damage. Found in poultry, seafood, organ meats, whole-grain products, onions, garlic, and mushrooms.

Sodium - With potassium, regulates the body's fluid balance; promotes proper muscle function. Found in table salt, dairy products, seafood, seasonings, and most processed foods.

Sulfur - Component of two essential amino acids in protein foods.

Zinc - Next to iron, zinc is the second most abundant trace mineral in the body. It is important in enzyme activity needed for cell division, growth and repair of wounds, and a strong immune system. Zinc also affects taste and smell, the metabolism of carbohydrates, the replication of DNA, and helps immune system fight microbes. Found in seafood (especially oysters), meat, liver, eggs, milk, brewer's yeast, whole wheat bread, and wheat germ.

Multiple Sclerosis. A degenerative disease of the central nervous system in which hardening of tissue occurs throughout the brain or spinal cord or both.

Myopia. Blurred long distance vision.

Niacin. Nicotinic acid, one of the B vitamins in living cells essential for growth.

Nitrates. Free radicals as a salt or ester of nitric acid, which can attack cells and cause cancer.

Nucleic Acid. Found in all living cells, these complex linear compounds contain genetic information.

Pantothenic Acid. A component of the vitamin B complex, common in liver, but found in all living tissue.

pH. A measure of the acidity or alkalinity of a solution, numerically equal to 7 for neutral solutions. The number gets larger with increasing alkalinity and smaller with increasing acidity.

Phagocytosis. The envelopment and digestion of bacteria or other foreign bodies by phagocytes.

Phytochemicals. Substances in fruits and vegetables that seem to protect against cancer and other degenerative diseases.

Platelet Aggregation. Clotting of blood.

Polyphenols. Strong antioxidants found in foods such as green tea.

Polysaccharides. A group of nine or more monosaccharides joined by glycosidic bonds such as starch and cellulose.

Proanthocyanadins (PCOs). A subgroup of polyphenols that are antioxidant flavonoids.

Prostaglandins. Hormones which if overactive can cause hypertension, cancer, asthma, and excessive blood clotting. Garlic keeps prostaglandins in check producing normal, healthy hormone levels.

Protein. Any of a group of complex nitrogenous organic compounds of high molecular weight that contain amino acids as their basic structural units and that occur in all living matter and are essential for growth and repair of animal tissue.

Qi. Asian word for life force in all living things.

Quercitin. Antioxidant phytochemical that inhibits cellular mutation, carcinogens, clot formation, and inflammation. Found in grape skins, red and white wine.

RE. Retinol Equivalent measurement for Vitamin A in animal or plant sources. See IU.

Retinol. A weaker version of the vitamin A cream, retinoic acid, approved by the Food and Drug Administration to reduce fine lines and wrinkles and skin discolorations associated with aging.

Riboflavin. A crystalline orange-yellow pigment that is the principal growth-promoting factor in the vitamin B2 complex, found in milk, leafy vegetables, fresh meat, egg yolks, and produced synthetically. Also called "lactoflavin."

Saturated Fats. Lipids that are usually solid at room temperature and tend to raise total blood cholesterol levels.

Silymarin. An antioxidant flavonoid in milk thistle that helps protect the liver by provoking increased production of two human body antioxidants: glutathione and superoxide dismutase.

Spirulina. Blue-green algae.

Superoxide Dismutase. A strong antioxidant produced by the liver.

T-Cells. T4 lymphocytes are immune cells that help trap and control foreign cells in the body. The AIDS virus attaches to T-cells, which interferes with the body's defense system and causes weakness and vulnerability to other diseases that can kill.

Terpenes. Antioxidant phytochemicals that stimulate anticancer enzymes. Found in citrus fruits.

Tinnitus. Ringing in the ears. Can be temporary or chronic. Aspirin and other drugs can cause tinnitus if used in high doses for long periods.

Unsaturated Fats. Liquid at room temperature; less likely than saturated fats to build up plaque in blood circulation system.

Vitamins:

A - Retinols. Improve night vision; needed for growth and cell development; maintain healthy skin, hair, nails, gums, glands, bones, and teeth; may help prevent lung cancer. Found in animal products and the beta-carotene of orange and yellow fruits and vegetables such as carrots, squash, cantaloupes, and in leafy green vegetables.

B1/Thiamine. Necessary for healthy energy metabolism and to maintain normal digestion, appetite, and proper nerve function. Found in pork, legumes, nuts, seeds, grains, and fortified cereals.

B2/Riboflavin. Essential for energy metabolism and healthy adrenal function. Found in fortified cereals and grains; lean meat and poultry; milk and other dairy products; raw mushrooms.

B3/Niacin. Needed for energy metabolism and normal growth. Large doses can lower cholesterol. Found in lean meats, poultry, seafood, milk, eggs, legumes, cereals, and fortified breads.

B5/Pantothenic Acid. Helps energy metabolism and normalizes blood sugar levels; synthesizes antibodies, cholesterol, hemoglobin, and some hormones. Found in almost all foods.

B6/Pyridoxine. Aids metabolism of proteins, carbohydrates, and energy release; proper nerve function; synthesis of red blood cells. Found in meat, fish, poultry, grains, cereals, green leafy vegetables, potatoes, and soybeans.

B12/Cobalamins. Needed to make red blood cells, DNA, RNA, and myelin for nerve fibers. Found in animal products from meat to dairy.

C/Ascorbic Acid. Strengthens blood vessel walls; helps iron absorption and healing; aids sustaining more normal blood cholesterol levels which counteracts atherosclerosis. Found in many fruits, citrus fruits and juices, melons, berries, and many vegetables including peppers, broccoli, and potatoes.

D/Calciterol. Necessary for calcium absorption; helps build and maintain strong bones and teeth. Found in fortified milk and butter, egg yolks, fatty fish, fish liver oils, and is made by the human body when exposed to sunshine.

E/Tocopherols. An important antioxidant that protects fatty acids; maintains muscles and red blood cells. Found in eggs, vegetable oils, margarine, mayonnaise, nuts and seeds, fortified cereals, and green leafy vegetables.

K. Essential for normal blood clotting. Found in spinach, cabbage, other green leafy vegetables, pork, liver, and green tea.

Biotin. Aids energy metabolism. Found in egg yolks, soybeans, cereals, and yeast.

Folate/Folic Acid. Needed to make DNA, RNA, and red blood cells and to synthesize certain amino acids. Found in liver, yeast, broccoli, other cruciferous vegetables, avocados, legumes, and many raw vegetables.

Miracle SUPER FOODS That Heal

Bibliography

ABRAMS, Karl J. *Algae to the Rescue!* Logan House Publications, 1996.

ANDERSON, Jean and Barbara Deskins, Ph.D., R.D. *The Nutrition Bible.* William Morrow and Co., New York, 1995.

BALCH, James, M. D. *The Super Antioxidants.* M. Evans and Co., 1998.

BELING, Stephanie, M.D. *Power Foods.* HarperCollins Publishers, 1997.

BERGNER, Paul. *The Healing Power of Echinacea and Goldenseal and Other Immune System Herbs.* Prima Publishing, 1997.

BEWICKE, Dyhana and Beverly Potter. *Chlorella: The Emerald Food.* Ronin Publishing, 1984.

ELKINS, Rita. *Blue-Green Algae, Spirulina and Chlorella: The Tonifying, Nutritive, Detoxifying Green Wonderfoods.* Woodland Publishing, 1996; and *Bilberry-Natural Enhancement for Visual and Cardiovascular Health.* Woodland Publishing, 1996.

FULDER, Stephen, Ph.D. *The Book of Ginseng and Other Chinese Herbs for Vitality.* Inner Traditions International, Ltd., 1993.

HOBBS, Christopher. *Milk Thistle: The Liver Herb.* Botanica, 1993.

JENSEN, Bernard, Ph.D. *Bee Well, Bee Wise.* Bernard Jensen Publisher, 1994.

Miracle SUPER FOODS That Heal

KAPOOR, L. D. *Handbook of Ayurvedic Medicinal Plants*. CRC Press, Boca Raton, Florida, 1990.

KEVILLE, Kathi. *Ginseng*. Keats Publishing, 1996.

LaCHANCE, Paul. *Nutraceuticals-Designer Foods III: Garlic, Soy and Licorice*. Food and Nutrition Press, 1997.

LAUX, M. Cures from the Rain Forest. Phillips Publishing, Potomac, Md, 1995.

LEE, William R. *Kelp Dulse and Other Supplements from the Sea*. Keats Publishing, 1983.

LIEBERMAN, Shari, Ph.D. *The Real Vitamin and Mineral Book*. 2nd Ed., Avery Pub. Group, Garden City Park, N. Y., 1997.

MANNINE, Betsy Russell. *Wheatgrass Juice, Gift of Nature*. Greensward Press, 1992.

MINDELL, Earl, R.Ph., Ph.D. *Herb Bible*. Simon & Schuster, 1992; and *Earl Mindell's Supplement Bible*. Fireside, 1998.

MITSCHER, Lester A., Ph.D., and Victoria Dolby. *The Green Tea Book, China's Fountain of Youth*. Avery Publishing Group, 1998.

MOSS, Ralph W., Ph.D. Cancer Therapy, pages 153-159. Equinox Press, New York, 1994.

MURRAY, Frank. *Ginkgo Biloba: Therapeutic and Antioxidant Properties of the Tree of Health*. Keats Publishing, 1996.

MURRAY, Michael, N.D. and Joseph Pizzorno, N.D. *Encyclopedia of Natural Medicine*. Prima Publishing, 1990.

PAPAS, Andreas and Jean Carper. *The Vitamin E Factor: The Miraculous Antioxidant for the Prevention and Treatment of Cancer, Heart Disease and Aging*. Harper Collins, 1999.

PASSWATER, Richard. *The Friendly Bacteria*. Keats Publishing, 1988.

POLUNIN, Miriam. *Healing Foods*. D. K. Publishing, Inc., 1997.

SEIBOLD, Ronald L. *Cereal Grass: Nature's Greatest Gift*. Keats Publishing, 1994.

STEENBLOCK, David, D. O. *Chlorella*. Aging Research Institute, Mission Viejo, Ca., 1996.

TENNEY, Louise, M. H. *Today's Herbal Health*, pages 75-76; 136. Woodland Books, Third Edition, 1992.

ULRICH, Gail. *Herbs to Boost Immunity: Herbal Tonics to Keep You Healthy and Strong, Including Echinacea, Siberian Ginseng, Astragalus and More*. Keats Publishing, 1997.

WADE, Carlson. *Health from the Hive: Honey...Bee Pollen...Bee Propolis...Royal Jelly*. Keats Publishing, 1992.

WERBACH, Melvyn, M.D. and Michael Murray, N. D. *Botanical Influences on Illness*. Third Line Press, 1994.

WICHTL, M. *Herbal Drugs and Phytopharmaceuticals: A Handbook for Practice on a Scientific Basis*. Medpharm Scientific Publishers, Stuttgart, Germany, 1995.

WIGMORE, Ann, N. D. *The Sprouting Book*. Avery Publishing Group, 1986; and *Why Suffer?* Ann Wigmore Foundation, 1986.

References

Cadoux, Deb and Alex, M.D.
Greenspring Rejuvenation Center
6884 East Sunrise Drive
Tucson, Arizona 85750
Tel: 520-529-9665
Fax: 520-529-9669
Santa Monica, Ca.: 310-260-3293
Anti-Aging and Longevity Medicine

Cymerint, Mark, D. C.
25571 Marguerite Parkway
Suite 2M
Mission Viejo, Calif. 92692
Tel: 949-707-5785

Gauthier, Patricia
Tel: 310-312-9684
Service: Massage Therapy, Dermal Technician, Skin Rejuvenation

Ghaly, Fouad I., M. D.
3655 Lomita Blvd., # 205
Torrance, Calif. 90505
Tel: 310-375-5926

La Perla, Pearl, A.M.D.
1006 Manor Drive
Reno, Nevada 89509
Tel: 775-348-6004
Ayurvedic Healing

Naugle, Mili, M.A., MFCC
1225 Entrada Glen
Escondido, Calif. 92027
Tel: 760-746-8646
E-mail: Mili54@home.com
Psychotherapy and Nutritional Healing

Page, Chris
Tel: 213-748-2261
E-mail: chrisnotes@aol.com
Products: Music composition for movies and television.

Rubens, Laurent, D. C.
Bayside Wellness Center
2634 Wilshire Blvd.
Santa Monica, Calif. 90403
Tel: 310-315-1828

Index

A

Acerola 13, 15-16, 68

Acetylcholine 43

Acid 60

Acidophilus 48-49

Acne 33, 61

Adaptation to darkness 25

Adaptogen 21, 58-59

Adenosine Triphosphate (ATP) 54

Adrenal glands and hormones 45

Age spots 45

Aging 22, 35, 38, 41

AIDS 58

Albumin 27-28

Alcohol 10, 14, 28, 43, 46, 54

Alfalfa 17, 27, 68

Algae, chlorella and spirulina 27-28, 56-57

Alkaline 14, 60

Allantoin 58

Allergies 23, 26, 28, 33, 35, 57

Almonds 29

Alzheimer's disease 34-35

Amanita mushrooms 46

American Medical Association 5, 32

Amino acids 14, 23, 26, 40, 50, 57, 59

Anemia 23, 57-58

Anger or fear 10

Anthocyanosides 25

Anti-inflammatory 32-33

Miracle SUPER FOODS That Heal

Antibacterial 15, 33, 50

Antibiotics 10, 33, 48-50

Antihistamine 23

Antimicrobial 48

Antioxidants 8-9, 14, 16, 22-27, 34-41, 46, 54, 56, 63

Antiviral 15

Apple pectin and fiber 18-19, 68

Apricots 24

Arame seaweed 31

Arteries 24, 30, 37

Arteriosclerosis 45, 54

Arthritis 15, 22, 33, 37, 44-45, 54, 61

Artificial coloring 10

Asia 26, 39, 44, 52

Aspartic acid 40, 50

Asthma 28, 35

Astragalus root 20-21, 68

Alantic seaweed 31

Attention Deficit Disorder (ADD) 4, 35

B

B vitamins See Vitamins

Bacteria 17, 21, 31, 41, 48

Bad Breath 49

Barbecued meats 36

Bark of pine trees 36

Barley grass 19, 22, 68

Bee pollen 23, 68

Beet juice 24, 68

Beta-carotene 12, 17, 22-24, 27, 56, 61

Beta-ecdysone 58

Betaine 17

Bi-polar molecules 42

Bilberry 25, 68

Bile acids 18

Bioflavonoid 16, 46

Biotin 44, 50, 53

Miracle SUPER FOODS That Heal

Carcinogens 22, 40, 48

Cardiovascular disease 24, 37, 41

Carotene 61

Carotenoids 24

Carper, Jean 31

Carrots 24, 56, 61

Cartier, Jacques 36

Cartilage 37

Casein 14

Catalase 63

Catechins 39-41, 68

Cell damage 22, 29, 34

Cell growth 24, 42, 46

Central nervous system 55

Cerebral hemorrhage 23

Cerebrovascular 35

Chemical poisoning 57

Chemical preservatives 10

Chemotherapy 20-21, 40

China 34, 40, 44, 52, 54

Chinese medicine 18, 20, 44, 54

Chlorella 27-28, 68

Chloroform 37

Chlorophyll 17, 22, 27, 56-57, 60-62

Cholesterol 15, 18-19, 22, 26, 30, 37, 42, 48-49, 54, 58

Choline 42-43

Chromium 41, 44

Chronic fatigue 21, 28, 53, 56

Cigarettes 10

Cincinnati, Ohio 32

Circulatory system 25, 32, 45-46, 58

Cirrhosis 46

Co-enzymes 23

Cobalt 27, 61

Colds 15, 21, 32-33, 45

Colitis 23

Collagen 37

Miracle SUPER FOODS That Heal

Colon 14, 16-18, 22, 41, 49

Constipation 23, 31, 44, 61

Copper 22, 27, 31, 41, 50, 53, 59

Corinthians II 9:6 1

Corn 14, 42

Corticosteroids 48, 53

Culpepper 46

Cymerint, Mark A. viii

Cysts 30

D

D-Alpha Tocopherol Acetate (vitamin E) 29-30, 68

Dairy 48

Dandruff 61

Depression 54

Dermis 37

Detoxify 17, 27, 41, 47, 55, 57, 59, 61

Diabetes 37, 41, 49, 54-55, 57, 59

Diabetic retinopathy 37

Diarrhea 20, 49

"Diet, Nutrition and Cancer Status" 61

Digestive tract 6, 26, 41, 48-49, 59, 61

DNA 8, 27, 34, 40-41, 63

Dolby, Victoria 41

Drugs 28, 43, 45

Dulse 31, 68

Dwarf ginseng 52

Dyes 14

E

E. coli 48

Ears 6, 35

Echinacea angustifolia 32-33, 68

Eczema 33, 61

Eggs 29, 42, 61

Elasticin 37

Eleutherococcus senticosus 52-55

Eleutherosides 52

F

Folacin 63

Folic acid 50

Framingham, Massachusetts 9

France 37

Free radicals 8-9, 22, 25, 30, 33-34, 36-37, 40-41, 46, 54, 56-58, 63

Friendly bacteria 49

Fungus 34, 48

G

Gallic esters 37

Gamma globulin 50

Gastrointestinal 23-24, 57

Gastric ulcers 45

Genesis 1:29 vi

German 32, 46, 53

Germanium 59

Ginkgo biloba 34-35, 68

Ginkgoales 34

Ginkgolides 35

Ginseng 53-54

Ginsenosides 53

Glucomannan root powder 44-45, 68

Glucose 35

Glutamic acid 40

Glutamine 40

Glutathione 46

Glutathione peroxidase 9, 63

Gluten 14, 26

Glycogen 56

Glycosides 45

Glycyrrhizic acid 44

Goldenseal 33

Gram 12

Grape-seed extract 10, 36-38

Greece 44, 60

Green foods 9, 17, 29, 60

Green tea 10, 28, 39-41, 68

Miracle SUPER FOODS That Heal

K

Kelp 31

Kenya, Africa 49

Kidney stones 32, 61

Kombu seaweed 31

Kona, Hiwaii 57

L

Lactase enzymes 48

Lacteals 6

Lactic acid 48-49, 54

Lactobacilli 49

Lactose 48

Lady Thistle 46

Laugh 10

Laxatives 18

Lead 4

Lecithin 15, 23, 37, 42-44, 68

Leg and arm cramps 30

Leukemia 61

Leukocytes 53

Leukotrienes 47

Lick weed 44

Licorice root 44-45, 68

Life expectancy 15, 48, 52

Ligaments 37

Lignan phytochemicals 22

Lipid peroxidation 34

Liposomes 19

Lithium 31

Liver 21-22, 27-28, 40-42, 45-46, 49, 54, 57-58, 63

Lloyd brothers 32

Los Angeles, Ca. 38

Love 10

Low cancer rate 28

Lowering cholesterol 28, 31

Lungs 17, 28-30, 39-40, 45, 53, 61

N

O

Oxygen bars 7

P

Pain 53

Paleozoic era 34

Panax 52-55

Panaxosides 53

Pancreas 40, 56

Pantothenic acid 44, 50, 53

Papayas 24

Parasites 4, 18

Passwater, Richard, Ph.D. 57

Pasteur Institute 48

Pathogens 48-49

Patrick, Jay 15

Pauling, Linus 15

Pawnee City, Nebraska 32

PCBs 28

PCOs 37

Pen Tsao ching 52

Permian 34

Pesticides 4, 7, 28

Pfaffosides 58

pH 16, 60

Phagocytosis 28

Pharyngeal glands 50

Phenylalanine 57

Phosphatidylcholine 37

Phospholipid 42

Phosphorous 7, 17, 22, 27, 41-44, 50, 59, 61

Phytochemicals 58

Phytonutrients 9

Phytosterols 45, 58

Pine bark 37

Plaque 41

Plasma 42

Platelet aggregation 30

Pollen 23

Polyphenols 40

Polysaccharides 20, 33, 56

Poor circulation 35

Portuguese 58

Potassium 17, 22, 26-27, 31, 41, 45, 50, 59, 61

Poultice of green tea leaves 41

Prayers 11

Pregnant 21, 35, 41, 47, 54

Pre-menstrual syndrome 30

Preservatives 14

Proanthocyanadins (PCOs) 36-37

Probiotic culture 48-49, 68

Processed foods 36, 40

Proline 40

Prostate 40

Proteins 9-10, 17, 23, 37, 49-50, 56, 58, 63

Psalm 24:1 13

Psoriasis 33, 61

Purple Coneflower 32

Pyorrhea 61

Q
Qi 20

Queen bees 50-51

Quercitin 16, 39

Quiroga, H., Ph.D. 54

R
Radiation 4, 9-10, 21, 23, 28, 40, 54, 57, 61

Rectal 23

Red blood cells 29, 47

Red ginseng 55

Reproductive aid 29

Retinol Equivalent (RE) 12

Retinal purple 25

Rhamnose 56

Miracle SUPER FOODS That Heal

Miracle SUPER FOODS That Heal

.

About the Author

Tony O'Donnell is a Doctor of Naturopathy certified in Neurolinguistic Programming (N.L.P.). He is also a certified hypnotherapist and nutritionist who speaks before West Coast audiences. He is the founder and president of one of the most innovative health and nutrition companies on the market today, which produces Emerald Greens, "America's favorite superfood." In 2001, he was honored by both the Leukemia Society and Angels on Earth Foundation as their "Man of the Year."

Dr. O'Donnell was born into a family of eleven children in Donegal, Ireland. When he was twenty-one, his father died of heart disease. Four other family members, including his fiancée, passed on after battles with cancer. These traumatic experiences motivated Tony to take charge of his own health and to help others lead healthier lives. Tony's mission is to love, care, share, and help others understand quality living.

Dr. O'Donnell graduated from the University College in Galway, Ireland and later studied at the British Homeopathic College and the University of Devonshore, where he received his degree as a Doctor of Naturopathy. He is also a certified herbalist and nutritionist.

In Ireland, Dr. O'Donnell hosted several radio shows. Today in the United States, he is heard daily on 1,000 radio stations across the country speaking about natural health. In addition to radio, he has been interviewed extensively on ABC, CBS, and FOX television networks and is the featured Naturopathic Doctor on ABC-TV, Phoenix.

For five years, Dr. O'Donnell was vice president of a major nutritional corporation and formulated twenty leading vitamin products, including the top seller Emerald Greens. He is single and resides in Santa Monica, California. His greatest joy is helping others to achieve abundant health.

Miracle SUPER FOODS That Heal

If you would like to write me with any questions, comments or suggestions, I would love to hear from you. Please send all correspondence to:

Attn: Dr. Tony O'Donnell, N. D.
O'Donnell's Health Advantage, Inc.
1148 Fourth Street, Suite 115-116
Santa Monica, California 90403
Tel: 310-458-1169
Fax: 310-458-9450

Website: http://www.emeraldgreens.com
E-mail: Doctony@earthlink.net